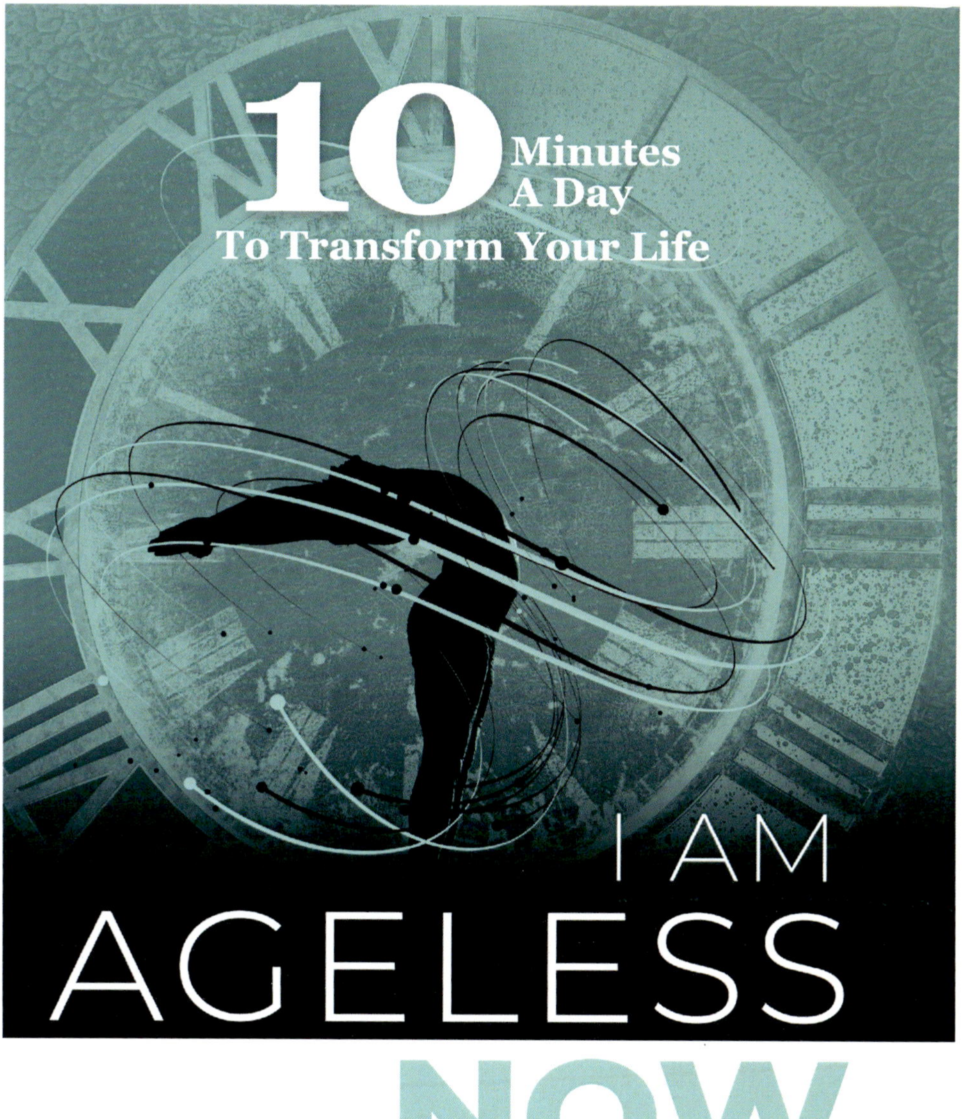

10 Minutes A Day To Transform Your Life

I AM AGELESS NOW

LESLEE BENDER | MELODY MARLER

Printed in the United States of America
ISBN: 978-1-951610-06-7
I Am Ageless Now / Leslee Bender & Melody Marler/1st ed., November 2020
www.iamagelessnow.com

Train your brain to love movement
It all begins with your mindset.

Part 1
Massage, Fascia, Posture

Part 2
Mindfulness

Part 3
Mindful Eating for Ageless Now Health

Part 4
Movement

Part 5
30-day Ageless Now Transformation

The I Am Ageless Now Collaboration

We met while waterskiing at a lake in Orlando. Both of us are Baby Boomers and have a similar philosophy about staying active and ageless. We had both recently found great guys (both of whom are a bit younger than us), who share our love for waterskiing and being active. We are conscious about how we eat and live, and are living our best lives. Neither one of us feels the need to be over-enhanced cosmetically and are comfortable in our skin.

Chronologically we are Boomers, but with respect to aging physically, we act and feel much younger. If you've wondered about how you can become more active and flexible, or feel less pain in your body, take a look at how to live agelessly, in the now. It does require effort, but you don't have to beat the heck out of your body at a gym or in a boot camp-type class. (In fact, please don't do that! For the actively aging population, extreme workouts can cause more harm than good.)

Today, unfortunately, many people sit for a majority of the day in a cubicle, at a desk, or in a car. You'll often see the phrase, "Sitting is the new smoking." Sitting for a long period of time compresses the spine and causes imbalances in the rest of the body's structure. This sedentary lifestyle creates a world of dysfunction from back and neck pain, and diabetes and obesity are often the result of this inactivity. When you sit for an extended period of time without moving, your muscles shorten, causing weakness, stiffness, and the inability to move correctly.

The Ageless Now lifestyle is built around science, but it's not scary or intimidating. And as you know (if you haven't been living under a rock), the latest available science changes with some frequency. Your doctor said chocolate is good for you? Yes, we like your doctor!

In fact, some of the things we grew up thinking were good for you (granola, dairy, bread) are actually the foods most people should avoid. Few medical folks advise people according to the latest science, so it's important for you to keep up with changes in that landscape on your own. The food pyramid most of us grew up with is a dense sandstorm of lies! Well, maybe it's not that bad. But you get the idea. Take it upon yourself to keep up. It's good for you—and interesting!

Rather than spending half your life in medical offices getting a constant stream of prescriptions, we advocate living a life full of activity, clean eating, sensible drinking, hydration, and mindful rest. You don't have to exercise like a Navy Seal recruit to have a healthy body. And stop worrying so much. That exacts a huge toll emotionally, but also on your physical body.

The best medicine? Indulge in simple pleasures like laughing, getting enough sleep, and eating good food, finding joy in good friends, family, and spending as much time as you can relaxing in nature. Do something you look forward to each day—something that lights you up. It goes a long way toward increasing your well-being. Our message of living the Ageless Now way is meant to provide you with health and happiness to live your best life for as long as you can.

Many workout programs today are based on very intense training for the "perfect body" without looking at the future negative consequences of damage and injury to the joints, tendons and ligaments due to improper posture, muscle imbalance, overuse, age, etc. Active Baby Boomers are walking examples of the need for hip and knee replacements due to not moving consistently, or overtraining improperly in their younger years.

That's why we wrote this book and created the movements in the I Am Ageless Now™ workout program. A strong, healthy, Ageless Now body is capable of carrying you through your life with flexibility and function, allowing you to do the things you love for your entire life. And the best part is, it's not difficult to start or sustain this way of living.

Aging happy and well, instead of sad and sick, is at least under some personal control. We have considerable control over our weight, our exercise, our education, and our abuse of cigarettes and alcohol... A successful old age may lie not so much in our stars and genes as in ourselves.

George E. Vaillant

Take care of your body.
It's the only place you
have to live.

Jim Rohn

INTRODUCTION

I Am Ageless Now

The **I Am Ageless Now Method** is a solution to living with less pain, more vitality, and a true solution to a better life. It's built around four essential components for your Ageless Now life:

MASSAGE to keep your fascia flexible.

MINDSET of positivity and gratitude, including strong motivation to become and stay ageless.

MINDFUL EATING for an ageless now body.

MOVEMENT to lubricate your joints.

Massage is well-known for its benefits, from stress reduction to pain management. When you massage the fascia, you allow it to become more lubricated and pliable, which will make your movement and exercise much more fluid and comfortable. Massaging before and after movement will increase blood flow, which in turns helps your muscles become stronger and efficient.

Mindset and motivation are key to living agelessly. When you think positive thoughts and are grateful for what your body can and will accomplish, you will reap the benefits of a longer, healthier, ageless life.

Take care with your thoughts; pay attention and catch yourself when you are sabotaging yourself. We suggest using mantras as you commit to living the Ageless Now way. A mantra is any positive statement that helps hold you in a mindset that contributes to your greater good. For example, while foam rolling your thighs, your mantra could be something like, "I am strong and stable and my legs carry me through any activity."

You have to set and make progress toward your goals to stay ageless. If you don't, you may physically deteriorate quickly. And you must have a passion for whatever it is to keep you ageless—a sport, hobby, staying active with family, or staying mobile to continue living on your own. When you set the intention, you have motivation. Even if your first goal is to massage your feet every day for five minutes or dedicate a portion of each day to slow down and meditate, it's a great start.

Mindful eating will help you develop an Ageless Now body. Being mindful helps you think about what you eat—how you fuel your body. You can make healthier food choices when you are mindful about what you choose to eat and how much you eat. Take it a step further by paying attention to all the sensations of each bite and savoring each bite by putting your fork down between bites. Mindful eating also includes paying attention to the nutrients your body needs to stay flexible and functional.

Movement is necessary for staying and remaining ageless. If you don't move or exercise regularly, your fascia becomes stuck, which leads to joint pain and dysfunction. This is why we have specific exercises you can easily follow for an Ageless Now body. Even starting these movements for just 10 minutes a day will make a huge difference in how you feel and move. When you add positivity with a daily mantra, the benefit is even more dramatic.

SO WHAT DOES IT MEAN TO BE AGELESS?

To be **ageless** is to live each and every day to the fullest, never looking back. The past is simply a lesson, and you don't have to keep repeating past mistakes or living the way you came to believe you were "supposed to" live. Whether you're in your 30s or your 80s or somewhere in between, you may have imposed limitations on yourself based on your current age. Or maybe you focus more on how you look and not so much on how you feel, or you think you're "too old" for certain activities.

Have you unintentionally abused your body? Maybe with the wrong diet or lack of movement? If you want to be around for a long time, for your friends, family AND yourself, and to live with less pain and more flexibility, it's time to pay attention. And it's not too late. Living the ageless way now is for everyone. And the best part is, you can start where you are.

Being ageless is not about aesthetics, and it's more than skincare. What really counts is how you live your life, and how you treat yourself and others.

Motivation is the key to success. You have to set and make progress toward your goals to stay ageless. If you don't, you can physically deteriorate quickly. It's important to understand **why** you want to stay active and ageless—whether it's for a sport, a hobby, to correct deteriorating health, or to stay active with family and friends. When you set an intention, you have motivation. Even if a goal is to massage your feet every day for five minutes or dedicate a portion of each day to slow down and meditate, it's a great start.

So how old are you anyway? What defines age to you? When most people think of aging, they immediately think of skin and topical creams or cosmetics. It's true that your skin is the largest organ of the body and often the first noticeable sign of an aging body. And while creams and cosmetics are important to many, it's what you put into your body and how you take care of it that has the greatest effect on your skin. We are bombarded with ads, magazines and social media telling us how we are supposed to look, with not a lot of focus on how we feel emotionally or physically. Anyone can be airbrushed or enhanced so they look good on film or publications, but they are still aging chronologically.

HOW YOU CAN LIVE AN AGELESS NOW LIFE

What can contribute the most to the aging process is a lack of discipline. We hear it time and time again: "I don't have the time or money to be healthy." Yes, you do! Do you take time to get your nails done? To treat yourself to sweets or other snacks because you've had a rough day? Or celebrate with pizza because you deserve it? Right?

It's easy to fall back on these "rewards." Our habits drive us, and it may have been ingrained in you over your lifetime that a reward is a sugary or salty fried snack. But you can make a different choice.

We live in a world of thousands and thousands of choices. Should we eat healthy food, or pop through the drive-through for a burger? Exercise, or surf stations on the TV and let mindless shows eat up our day? Take time to meditate or let the daily noise of conflict and drama dominate? When you take a moment to make the healthy choice, you'll realize it doesn't take much time to allow

Do not grow old, no matter how long you live. Never cease to stand like curious children before the great mystery into which we were born.

Albert Einstein

yourself to make a positive change. In a very short time, these choices will become subconscious actions and won't require as much in the way of decisions; they will become habits. And they all will help you defy aging.

GETTING STARTED: COMMIT TO A HEALTHIER, HAPPIER YOU

Set the stage for what you want to accomplish in a short amount of time. Think about how you feel physically and emotionally in your body. Then notice how you feel afterward!

What is it that you want to accomplish by changing your lifestyle to live an Ageless Now life? When you set the intention you have the motivation.

You can set an intention for:

- Stress reduction
- A new attitude
- Less pain
- Better flexibility
- Better focus
- Relaxation

Visualization IS necessary for change. When you start with a positive mindset, you'll be more present for whatever activity you are about to engage in. If you're starting a movement, for example, start with the idea that you can complete it even if you haven't been physically active in some time.

One of our favorite mantras is:

I now release and let go all thoughts and emotions, conscious and subconscious, that are not for my highest and best good. I am in the moment now. I am life inner-force energy now. I am relaxed. I am centered.

Here are some others you can use:
I am listening to my body now.
I am releasing all negativity from my body now.
I am letting go of my stress now.
I am letting the light shine in now.

Everyone has a choice in how they want to live. We hope that you too will make a decision to defy aging in every aspect of your life: body, mind and spirit.

It doesn't take a huge time commitment to change your life. But it may take a mindset shift. If you don't see yourself as an active person, you can change your thoughts about that, too. Everyone can make a choice to live the ageless way. Regardless of the shape you may have arrived at in midlife, one thing is certain: You are amazing and durable. Tiny steps made with commitment and habit will lead you to a lifestyle that can carry you through your years with agility and clarity.

But don't do it "someday." Do it now. It doesn't take several days or weeks or months to create a habit. **It takes just one decision.** Your decision. The time is NOW to be resilient, positive, active, mindful, happy—ageless. You can make the decision to start wherever you are and get up and move. Don't let life drive you. You're in the driver's seat, so take control NOW.

1
MASSAGE TO KEEP YOUR FASCIA FLEXIBLE

Strength that has effort in it is not what you need. You need the strength that is the result of ease.

Ida Rolfe

Skin, Skin, Skin! It's More Than Just Your Face

The skin is the largest organ in our body, and it's one of the most complicated. It's ever-changing, and it contains many cells and structures. The skin's primary function is to serve as a protective barrier that interacts with an environment that can be harsh at times—think brittle cold, heat, pollution, blazing sun. Our skin also helps regulate body temperature, sensing information from the surrounding environment (wind in your face, subzero wind chill), and plays an active role in our immune defenses, protecting the body from disease.

Learning how the skin functions begins with an understanding of the structure of the three layers of skin: the epidermis, the dermis, and subcutaneous. (Don't worry—we're not going to get all technical, and you don't have to dissect anything. And if you're wondering what on earth this has to do with massage, just hang tight. We're getting there.)

The epidermis is the outermost layer of the skin. Its thickness is different depending on where it is on your body. Your eyelids, for example, are much thinner than the soles of your feet. Humankind was designed that way for function. Our feet need a thicker layer of skin for absorption of the ground and gravity and for the multitude of tasks they perform, such as walking. The thicker skin lets our feet endure more friction.

The dermis is the middle layer of skin, which contains two important proteins that contribute to the skin's strength and texture: elastin and collagen. These two proteins keep your skin from wrinkling and sagging, but they break down with age, which is why you may recognize them from anti-aging product advertisements. The dermis also contains nerves, blood vessels, hair follicles and sweat glands. When you feel pain after you cut yourself, it's because of the nerves and receptors in your dermis.

The subcutaneous layer is made up of fat and collagen cells. This layer helps you retain heat, and it also absorbs shock and protects your internal organs from injury. If tissue in this layer begins to deteriorate, your skin may start to sag.

Voila! And there you have the aging process.

PROTECT THE SURFACE

There are many creams potions and lotions that are designed to protect your skin against the damaging effects of the sun. If you were part of the baby-oil-combined-with-iodine-tanning-club of past decades, you probably have skin damage. Tanning in the 60s, 70s and 80s was a thing, and many of those who overindulged in the rays now look like a Louis Vuitton suitcase. A touch of sun for a few minutes each day is actually good for you, but it's not good to bask for hours, especially now that the ozone layer has thinned out substantially. When you want to partake in outdoor activities, it's a no-brainer to properly protect yourself with high-level sunscreens.

COLLAGEN: FEEDING YOUR SKIN FROM THE INSIDE OUT

It seems like everyone is talking about collagen these days. It comes up a lot when people are talking about aging. Unfortunately, we do lose collagen as we age, and the collagen we make as we age is of a lower quality than it was when we were younger. Genetics also plays a part in how fast each person loses collagen.

Collagen is the most abundant protein in your body. It's one of the major building blocks of bones, skin, muscles, tendons, and ligaments. Collagen is also found in many other parts of the body, including blood vessels, corneas, and teeth. Think of it as the "glue" that holds all these things together. Collagen fibers give the body its shape and structure.

Besides aging, a number of factors come into play with collagen loss. Some other enemies of healthy skin are a poor diet (especially one high in sugar), being exposed to UV rays or pollution, and smoking. But it's not only skin that suffers as collagen levels drop. Lower collagen can also lead to joint pain, weaker muscles, and sometimes causes gastrointestinal issues as the lining in your digestive tract thins.

There are a multitude of collagen supplements on the market, including pills, powders, liquids and gelatin. These are often made from animals, which could be problematic for vegans and vegetarians. And as always, it's imperative to check with your doctor before trying any new supplements. One of the easiest ways to slow the aging process of your skin is to eat a diet full of collagen-rich nutrients. This allows you to take in more nutrients than you would by simply consuming collagen supplements.

Some collagen-rich foods include:

Dark leafy greens
Citrus fruits
Black and green olives
Flaxseeds and walnuts
Prunes
Tomatoes
Oysters
Fish, especially salmon
Red bell peppers
Bone broth
Berries
Lean beef
Eggs
Chicken
Legumes
Spirulina
Garlic
Cashews
Avocados

FASCIA: THE BODY'S PROTECTIVE COMPLEX WEB

All of us have experienced occasional lingering pain or discomfort, maybe a tightness we can't identify. Or maybe you've tried foam rolling or had a massage and marveled at how the pain you first

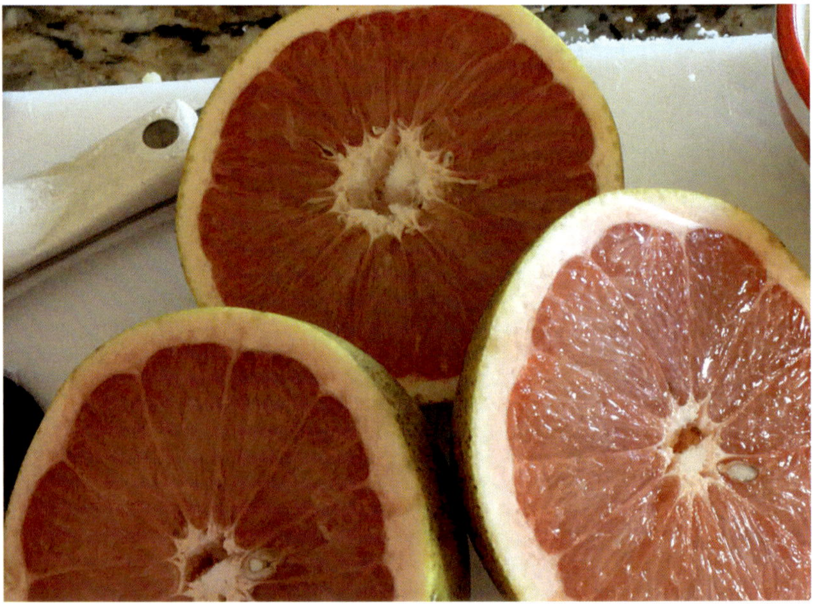

feel eventually gives way to relief. The relief you're feeling comes from loosening your fascia, the internal connective tissue that wraps around our organs, holding the parts together and providing support.

Fascia is made mostly of collagen, and provides a supportive and movable wrapping like a web for nerves and blood vessels as they pass through and between muscles. It provides stability and motion and minimizes the stress on the spine and permits the muscles to function as they should. Without it, the body would have no stability or muscle strength. It supports the entire skeletal system, and without it we would not have structure.

Think of fascia as being similar to the white fibrous membrane of a grapefruit, just under the peel. This analogy illustrates the way the fascia holds things together internally.

SO, CAN I REPAIR DAMAGED FASCIA?

What the grapefruit analogy doesn't really explain well is the function fascia plays in supporting a healthy body. If you are engaging in a physical activity and get hurt, for example, the structure of the fascia works as a shock absorber for the impact. So while it will tighten up due to the impact of the injury, the good news is, you can also reverse the damage to your fascia. The keys are hydration and motion. So really, you can also think of fascia like a sponge. While it's hydrated, you can do all sorts of things to it—wring it out, twist it into a spiral, fold it in half—and it will return to its original shape. Dry it out, however, and you've got a whole other scenario, one of immobility, muscle tightness, and possibly pain.

Drinking plenty of water and paying attention to soft tissue work (massage) will help you repair any damage to your fascia. You don't

Wisdom is valuable. You've earned it with your experience. Age is the advantage. We are the difference-makers.

have to get a professional massage every day—although, would anyone really complain about that?

There are a number of self-massage routines you can do using a simple tennis ball and/or a foam roller. You'll find those in the chapter on movement. There's a reason most of the routines begin with rolling out your feet. It's one of the most sensitive areas of our bodies, and one of the most neglected. Loosening up your fascia in your feet and everywhere else, for that matter, will also help you move better as you begin your I Am Ageless Now movements. It warms up your muscles as it keeps your fascia moving. If you take care of your fascia, you will be amazed at your increased flexibility and movement.

And of course, we always recommend treating yourself to a professional massage! You know you deserve it.

WHAT ABOUT MY SCAR?

When you cut yourself and it forms a scar, think of the scar as glue. When you don't manipulate the glue, it doesn't move. Scar creams work, but you also have to massage that area. Scar tissue can be really deep, and if it isn't manipulated, you won't have movement. Depending on the injury, consult with your physician as to when it's safe to have therapy done on a scar.

FASCIA AND YOUR POSTURE

Poor posture affects fascia, and unhealthy fascia affects posture. Over time, incorrect posture can form tightened/hardened fascia in particular areas, which further upsets the natural, neutral alignment of your spine and skeletal system.

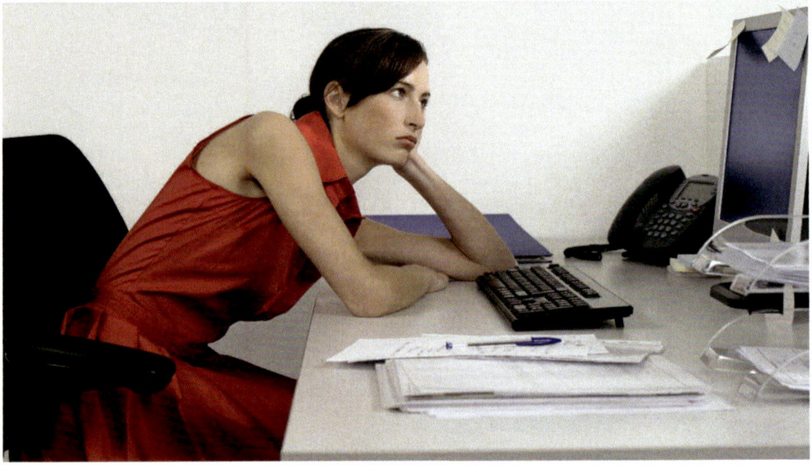

This can be seen by those who sit slouched in front of a computer, phone or table, as well as in those who stand for prolonged periods of time without awareness of their postures. A slouched position causes considerable stress on the discs and ligaments of the lower back, weakens the muscles in the hamstrings and glutes, creates a tightening of the abdominal muscles, and over time increases the hardened fascia in the abdominal area.

Once you are in this slouched position over a computer or couch, your fascia molds to your habits. This positioning continues to contribute to a hunchback posture, as the skeletal system is pulled forward into an unnatural bend. This also adds to the aging process.

In addition to poor posture and improper training techniques, fascia can also become tightened due to trauma, chronic strain, immobility, dehydration, and emotional stress. In addition to immobility and inflammation, unhealthy fascia has been linked to depression, tinnitus and lack of concentration.

Your posture defines you! If you walk into a room like you own it, with your shoulders back and your head held high, you are the picture of what defying the aging process looks like. Have you seen

Jane Fonda lately? In her eighties her posture and carriage defines a much younger woman.

When you hold yourself in good posture you not only take a lot of pressure off your spine, you will also look much younger and healthier. Too much of our time is spent sitting over cell phones or tablets or computers all day, and then we wonder why our backs hurt and our shoulders are becoming hunched. This is one area where you need to be diligent until you build a subconscious habit of simply sitting up straight and holding your shoulders in good posture.

Better yet, put the phone or computer mouse down and go for a walk. Detaching from screens is a huge way to increase your well-being. Cell phones obviously play a huge role in the world today, but sometimes they can dominate our lives in a negative way. If you work at a computer screen, make sure you build in time for screen breaks, and get up and move.

Some simple steps to hold yourself in good posture: Engage your core, lengthen your spine by standing tall, hold your head up and imagine you are walking proudly onto a stage. You will look AND feel better.

ESSENTIALS OF AGELESS ALIGNMENT

Your alignment is essential when exercising. For example, a lot of people sit primarily throughout their day. As we mentioned before, this can create poor posture. Let's look at the alignment of your spine. Neutral is where your spine is held in place symmetrically. Your spine is meant to be vertical with the natural curvatures. When you have good posture and alignment you use less energy in activities and will most likely have less back pain.

When you hold yourself in good ageless alignment you have more confidence and self-esteem. Try standing tall and see how it feels from the ground up. Take notice of how you feel in your body when you are taller both mentally and physically. Now position yourself into a slouch. See how that feels in your body? And what did it do to your mindset? Slouching is often synonymous with aging, and it actually does age your spine by compressing it.

MASSAGE: MOTION IS LOTION

One of the simplest and best things to do every day as you brush your teeth is to massage your feet with a tennis ball. Giving your feet a dose of reflexology first thing in the morning will help you keep your fascia healthy and, at the same time, increase your energy for the day.

Reflexology rests on the ancient Chinese belief in qi or ch'i (pronounced "chee"), or "vital energy." According to this belief, qi flows through each person. When a person feels stressed, their body blocks qi, which can age us. It can also cause an imbalance in the body that leads to illness. Reflexology aims to keep qi flowing through the body, keeping it balanced and disease-free.

In Chinese medicine, different body parts correspond with different pressure points on the feet. Using a tennis ball to address pressure to various parts of the foot will not duplicate work by a therapist or reflexologist, but you can still self-treat areas that correspond with direct relationship to your fascia for quick results. Touch can send energy flowing through a person's body until it reaches the area in need of healing. This is illustrated in the reflexology chart on the following page.

Foot Reflexology Chart

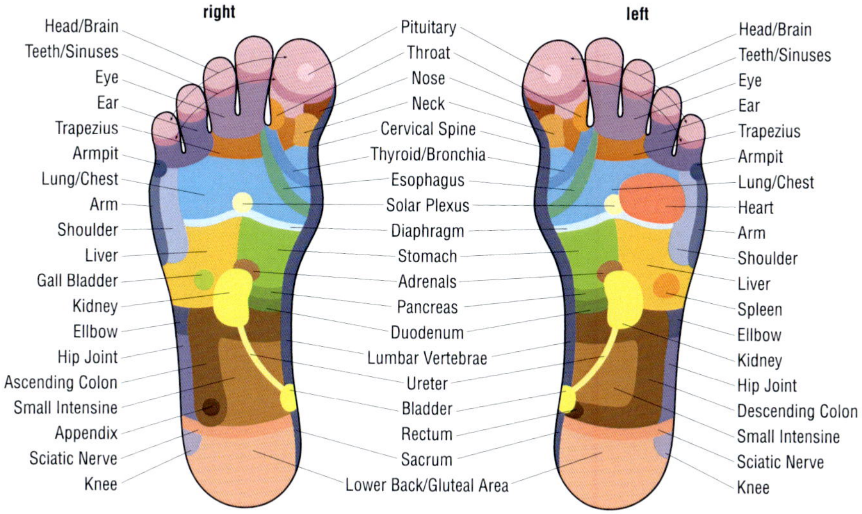

2
MINDSET OF POSITIVITY AND GRATITUDE

Stop acting as if life is a rehearsal. Live this day as if it were your last. The past is over and gone. The future is not guaranteed.

Wayne Dyer

The Influence of Your Thoughts

Our subconscious does not have a sense of humor. Keeping this in mind, if we think negatively about our body and the way it looks and feels, we will perpetuate our body looking and feeling in exactly that way. When you think positive thoughts and are grateful for what your body can and will accomplish you will reap the benefits of a longer, healthier, ageless life. Take care with your thoughts, pay attention and catch yourself when you are sabotaging yourself.

Here are a few examples of how you can change your thoughts from negative to positive:

Negative I am too fat and cannot change.
Positive I choose to be healthy.

Negative I am too tired all the time.
Positive I am abundantly full of energy.

Negative I am too old to do that.
Positive I am taking on a new adventure and loving it.

KNOWING YOUR EMOTION AND CHOOSING TO CHANGE

We all have "stuff." What are you dealing with emotionally? When you have a lot of negative emotion in your life, whether it's conscious or subconscious, it is often reflected in your posture and attitude. When you consciously reinforce positive emotions, you're more likely to physically and emotionally change.

Visualization is necessary for change. Make sure you set a positive stage to help you be present for the workout, and let your negative beliefs or emotions go for the time you are doing your movements and exercise. Listen to your body. Here are some others you can use:

I am releasing all negativity from my body.

I am letting go of my stress.

I am perfect.

I am light.

My body is my temple.

THOUGHTS ARE THINGS AND THEY HAVE WINGS

Mantras are intentional affirmations you repeat internally or aloud. With the I Am Ageless Now movements, we suggest using mantras throughout the movements to reinforce a positive mindset, especially if movement is new for you.

We have all had setbacks and self-doubts in life that have challenged our spirit. The human spirit fights to keep going no matter what the circumstance. Your negative thoughts are a habit, just like any bad habit, and the best way to get rid of a bad habit is to replace it with a good one. When a negative thought comes, nip it in the bud, tell it to take a seat, and think of something positive to put in its place. Keep doing this until it becomes a natural response.

Your own powerful, positive thoughts keep your mind focused, strong, and on task. Make sure you incorporate these thoughts throughout the movements you do this program.

Your own powerful, positive thoughts keep your mind focused, strong, and on task. Make sure you incorporate these thoughts throughout the movements you do with this program. Here are some to get you started:

I am fearless.

I am a miracle.

I am proud of my decisions.

I am amazing.

I am fortunate.

I am full of life.

I am in control of my thoughts, my mind, and my body.

I am magnificent.

I am safe and secure.

I am proud of who I am becoming.

I am abundant.

I am grateful.

I am free to learn, grow, and discover.

I am joyful.

I am trusting the journey.

I am willing to ask for help.

I am comfortable in my own skin.

I am strong.

I am desirable.

I am positive.

The secret of health for both mind and body is not to mourn for the past, worry about the future, or anticipate troubles, but to live in the present moment wisely and earnestly.

Buddha

I am courageous.

I am more than enough.

I am beautiful (handsome).

I am kind.

I am confident.

I am worthy of the blessings coming my way.

THE POWER OF THE NOW

There is power in living in the "now." It's why we named our book and program **I Am Ageless Now.** Right now, this very moment, is the now, the moment that matters—the one that can make the biggest difference. The past is over and the future isn't guaranteed. But today, this very moment, is.

Learning to live in the present moment gives you the power to live your best life. To live in the now means you are being conscious and aware, using all your senses. It means you aren't living in the past nor are you worrying about what the future will be. When you concentrate on being present, you focus your attention on the task at hand. You can give it your full attention, let go of the outcome, and make each moment more meaningful and valuable.

You still need to plan, set goals, and prepare for the future. But you can do all these things and still enjoy living in the moment. For instance, you may (we hope!) set a goal to exercise every day, increasing your flexibility and quality of life.

Too often we put enormous expectations on ourselves. We're always rushing to do this or finish that or hurrying to do something else. We never actually enjoy the process. We don't stop and think about where we are, so we miss the point of being there. When you live in the now, you learn to appreciate each moment and gather the lessons from each moment. It is living consciously, purposefully, and responsibly, and can make a huge contribution to living an Ageless Now lifestyle.

On the other hand, when we live in the past, hanging onto painful experiences, difficult times or wrongs we perceive were done to us, we are condemning ourselves to living the same now and in the future. Coming to terms with the past, knowing you can't change it, helps you move on. Living in the now means letting go of the past. It means you trust in the future, and you are more positive and optimistic in the present. You may begin to notice the beauty and wonder of the moment and the things around you, how to focus and manage your energy.

As you put it into practice, combining the movements and other essential components of living the Ageless Now way, you'll discover it's not as difficult as you may believe to make small changes that significantly improve your life.

BENEFITS OF AGELESS NOW MINDFUL LIVING

From improving your physical health to your mental status, being mindful enhances your life. By reducing stress and anxiety you are able to avoid the associated health consequences, such as high blood pressure, heart disease and obesity. Being mindful improves your psychological well-being as you become more in tune with what is happening around you. Most of us have been in a situation where you're with someone who is with you physically, but their mind is a million miles away and you can tell they are not mentally present. Maybe you've done this to others in the past. But when you make an effort to be fully present in the conversation, and ensure the other person is as well, you'll create a deeper connection and better communication.

When you are living in the moment, you are in better control over your mind, your body and your emotions. You are the one with the power to improve your life. For example, it's easier to see what needs to be done now instead of being overwhelmed by the scope of a large project and simply pushing it aside. You may find you are also more in tune with the world around you instead of being lost in your own thoughts all the time.

WHY LIVING IN THE MOMENT CAN BE A CHALLENGE

Even though there are many benefits of living in the moment, it can often be difficult to do. All our lives we've been encouraged to think about the future and remember the past. Advertising, notifications, messages, reminders, alerts are all geared to what's coming up or what happened previously. When we're constantly reminded of the past or thinking about the future, it can cause stress or anxiety. And, there is comfort in the possibility of what's to come, something that lies beyond today—hope. We have hope that tomorrow will be better than this moment, this now. So we are constantly thinking of what is next.

We don't worry about the present moment because it's already decided. That means our mind naturally goes to the past or to predicting the future. We use our past as the basis for what the future will be. This tendency can get out of control and we begin to see dangers that are not actually there.

Most people have a hard time staying focused on the moment. Our minds naturally wander. We have an innate ability to always be thinking, wandering, asking, pondering, and just having random thoughts. This is also why some people say they "can't" meditate. But it's a choice, just like choosing to be active and to eat nutritious food. We can change the tendencies of our brains. Practicing mindfulness makes it possible to overcome the harmful or destructive choices and make better ones.

HOW TO START LIVING IN THE MOMENT

You know that being mindful is important, but how do you start doing it? Here are some ways you can put mindfulness into practice.

- **Slow down**. Before beginning any activity, no matter what it is, take a deep breath and focus on the process.
- Make an effort to **live in the moment**. Make the commitment to begin changing your habits of rushing, not paying attention, and functioning by going through the motions. Notice where you are not being mindful.
- **Notice** when you find you aren't in the present moment. If you happen to be in a present moment that is stressful, notice how your thoughts and emotions affect your body. Turn your thoughts toward positivity to keep yourself in the now.
- **Engage** in what you are doing and enjoy the process. Train your mind to focus on your current activity. Stop worrying about tomorrow and realize tomorrow will happen no matter what. Redirect your mental energy into enjoying this moment.
- **Learn relaxation techniques** like meditation, deep breathing, and visualization, to help you stay calm.
- **Listen with attention** to your conversations, music—and the silence.

- **Notice** your surroundings. What do you see, hear, smell, feel?
- **Savor your food**. Chew slowly, enjoy the taste, and set your utensil down between bites.
- **Start each day with a smile.** Each day is full of possibilities. You can control your attitude every morning. Keep your attitude optimistic and intentional.
- **Be fully appreciative** of the moments of today—the sounds, sights, smells, the emotions you feel, the wins and the sorrows.
- **Let go** of past hurts and resentments. Choose to forgive and move on. When you forgive, it helps you more than anyone else. The person you forgive may not even be in this world anymore. Forgiveness doesn't mean the "wrong" was right. It just means you are releasing your hold on the negative memory. Often you're holding on to "wrongs" that were done years, maybe even decades, ago. Don't let this hurt and resentment color the rest of your life. Release it and see what joy can then be attracted into your life.
- **Love what you do.** If you just survive your work and are constantly waiting for the weekend to get here, you're wasting a good portion of your life. Either find a new job you enjoy or find things about your current career you can appreciate.
- **Listen to your body.** Your body will tell you if you are stressing, worrying, or not taking care of it.
- Think with **positivity and calm**.

- **Let go of outcomes.** When you live in the moment you don't stress or worry over how something will turn out. Take action, focus on the task, and let the outcome happen.

Learning to live in the now is an essential part of living a happy life. Start with one thing you can implement daily and work up to being present in every way.

BREATHING THE AGELESS NOW WAY

Have you ever worn one of the smart watches that pops you up every hour with a reminder to "take a minute to breathe"? We take it for granted, no doubt! It's subconscious for most.

While breathing usually occurs without much thought, it's also a necessary component of mindful living. Being mindful of your breath as you go through the movements in part 4 and fascial massage will not only make it easier, but it can also increase your lung capacity. Stronger lungs make everything more efficient.

When you breathe in air, blood cells receive oxygen and release carbon dioxide, a waste product that's carried back through your body and exhaled. Improper breathing can upset the oxygen and carbon dioxide exchange and contribute to anxiety, panic attacks, fatigue, and other physical and emotional disturbances.

Learning to breathe correctly will enhance everything you do. Practice taking a deep breath in and pause, then let it out. Do this about five times and notice how you feel! When you prepare to do one of the I Am Ageless Now movements, inhale through your nose and exhale through your mouth. Breathe deeply and slowly when doing the fascial massage in the movements section.

This type of breathing:

- Calms the mind, reducing worries and anxieties.

- Helps to focus on the movement and accomplish it more efficiently.
- Improves focus and attention, removing brain fog.
- Increases energy, enthusiasm and positivity.
- Boosts the immune system.
- Rejuvenates the body and mind.
- May slow down the aging process.

BREATHING EXERCISE

Sit still and close your eyes (this won't take long). Take a deep breath in through the nose and exhale somewhat forcefully out through your mouth. As you inhale feel the breath fill your belly. As you exhale, let your belly relax. Clear your mind for about three to five minutes and focus only on the sound and feeling of your breath.

THE BENEFITS OF ESSENTIAL OILS

When performing the massage movements and breathing exercises, we suggest you find an essential oil you like. There are many brands; make sure you choose one that is pure without any added chemicals. Before you begin the fascial massage movements, place a few drops of the oil on your wrists or hands, and rub them together. Hold your hands above your nose and breathe in the scent. This is meant to calm you and allow you to work not only with the physical benefit of massage, but to let go of any emotional blockages as well. As an added bonus, using an oil for energy when you exercise can also give you an extra boost. Some of the best oil scents for relaxation are lavender, ylang ylang, frankincense, vanilla, and citrus. For energy try orange, ginger, peppermint, bergamot, or lemon.

3
MINDFUL EATING FOR AGELESS NOW HEALTH

Nothing tastes as good as being alive feels.

Mindful Eating for An Ageless Now Body

A lot of us grew up mired in food myths (eat low-fat! granola is good for you!). We held food-centered activities, events, celebrations, and family gatherings. At the time, as a child, it felt wonderful. And right. Pretty much nothing about it sucked. But as we got older and realized things had to change, it became something to push against. We reward ourselves as if we're children when our lives as adults get too hard:

"I deserve licorice."

"I'm tired and all I want is a cookie and a glass of wine."

"I don't eat fast food that often. I'm stopping for a burger and fries."

How do these statements resonate with you? Following are a few questions about what you eat in any given week.

AGING EATING QUIZ

- How much white or wheat bread do you eat per week, other than 100% whole wheat?
- How many diet drinks or soda do you consume?
- How many energy boosting drinks with caffeine do you drink?
- How much red meat do you eat?
- How many processed foods do you eat (crackers, chips, cookies)?
- How many sandwiches with processed meat do you eat?
- How much candy do you eat?
- How much coffee do you drink? Do you add sugar and cream or creamer?
- How many times do you eat fast food?
- How much starch (pasta, rice, fries, etc.) do you eat?
- How much alcohol, including light beer or wine, do you drink?
- How often are you eating out?
- How much dairy do you consume?
- How many desserts do you consume?

You probably figured out where we're going with this. If you said you are consuming any of the above regularly you are on the path to aging. If you answered you consume more than one soda—even diet—you are aging.

If you are drinking energy drinks or similar products, drinking sugary drinks, eating processed food or sandwiches daily, stopping for fast food more than occasionally, craving sugar or caffeine, or consuming more than one alcoholic beverage per day—even "red wine in moderation"—you are aging.

Foods that will rob you of energy and age you: All processed meats, including sandwich meats, bacon and jerky; fast foods (hamburgers, fries, etc.); pizza; wings; ice cream; doughnuts; chips; artificial sweeteners; all processed food with high glycemic index (sugar); soft drinks, including diet soda; cookies, cakes, pies, candy; crackers; milk products; breads that are not 100% whole wheat; pasta.

You may be reading this and thinking to yourself, "Why yes, I eat this stuff. No wonder I feel like crap. And I am aging!" You can reverse the process, but you have to be willing to work, possibly give up some bad habits, and make healthier eating choices, if you want more energy and want to look and feel Ageless Now.

If you feel tired, bloated, or have pain in your joints, you are more than likely eating a diet that will age you. What if by changing one habit at a time you could add years to your life? Would you do it?

We make excuses every day and justify them with a vengeance. It can be something simple, like stopping for a burger instead of taking the time to pack a salad to take to work. If you're just "sort of" interested in changing your lifestyle, then you will age.

Excuses keep us from facing our fears. Are there unhealthy foods or drinks you think you just can't live without? It's so much easier to stay in our comfort zones than it is to change, and to change like your life depends on it. And guess what? Your life just might depend on you making a change.

EATING GOOD FOOD DOESN'T HAVE TO SUCK

So what should you eat? Everyone seems to have a take on what's "healthy." If you take a stroll through your favorite grocery store you'll see the produce section is often small and the bulk of the aisles are filled with prepared foods, full of added sugars and chemicals. No one is making this easy for us.

There's no one perfect diet, but there are some basic guidelines.

- Make half your plate fruits and vegetables.
- Keep your protein lean and unprocessed: Choose meats trimmed of fat, and eat seafood, beans, nuts, and seeds.
- Replace refined grains like white bread and white rice with whole grains like multigrain bread, brown rice, and oatmeal.
- Make sure the fats you eat are healthy. The aging brain desperately needs good fat. Not that long ago, fat was considered bad and everything became fat-free, which is, unfortunately, enhanced with sugar and other fillers.

EATING TOO MUCH SUGAR CAN AGE YOU

It's hard to dispute the fine taste of sugar. But in reality, it's like consuming the apple from the Adam & Eve story. If you're a label reader, you'll find sugar in many processed foods—some you would never expect. High fructose corn syrup is often used as a sugar substitute, and it's found in a huge number of products. Products like fat-free half and half are actually loaded with fillers (including high fructose corn syrup). Who knew?! The first step is to take great care when you're reading food labels.

Even if you aren't overweight, sugar can negatively impact your health. There are federal guidelines for limits on how much salt and saturated fat you should eat, but there doesn't seem to

Eat like you love
yourself.
Move like you love
yourself.
Speak like you love
yourself.
Act like you love
yourself.

Tara Stiles

be an upper limit on the recommended sugar intake. There's been a lot of recent research pointing to the harm sugar does to your cardiovascular system.

The American Heart Association isn't shy about its recommendation either, saying women should consume less than six teaspoons of added sugar and men less than nine teaspoons of added sugar per day. One can of sugar-sweetened soda would put all women and most men over that daily limit. Sugar also is 100% empty calories, with no fiber, vitamins, or any nutritional value whatsoever. And if you eat too much sugar, it can cause you to eliminate other healthier foods from your diet.

Those who study human fossils found no sign of cancer, diabetes or heart disease until humans started farming grains. And grains are used to make sugar. The bottom line is, sugar is poison. Some studies have claimed it's more addictive than heroin.

After you eat anything sugary and processed, your insulin peaks and your brain is screaming for more. Over-consumption of sugar is killing millions of people who are unaware of what they are doing. The body becomes so damaged, aged and unhealthy it no longer functions, and sometimes has to be managed with drugs. All of this can be avoided if we all eat to live, not live to eat.

WHAT ABOUT PROTEIN?

If you are a bodybuilder or high-end athlete then you are going to need more protein. The recommended daily amount is a daily intake of 0.8 grams per each Kg (1 Kg equals about 2.205 pounds) of body weight. For example if you are 196 pounds, then you would need 71 grams of protein per day. If you are 140 pounds, you need approximately 50 grams of protein per day.

We lose muscle mass every decade and muscle needs protein to keep lean and strong. The only way to fight muscle loss is to exercise, including some form of weight training, and consuming protein daily.

With a little extra effort, you can actually get enough plant-based protein. This also gives you a higher level of alkaline in your body, which fights diseases such as cancer. Organic green plants rich in nutrients and minerals such as spinach and kale will also have protein, but not enough. A single cup of fresh spinach, for example, contains less than 1 gram of protein per serving. A one-cup serving of spinach cooked in water contains 5.35 grams of protein—more because of the increased density per serving of the cooked spinach.

An average egg contains about 6 to 7 grams of protein depending on the size of the egg (a small egg has about 4.9 grams of protein, while a large egg contains 6.5 grams). Meat provides the most dense protein per serving. If you do eat meat, make sure it's lean and organic. Fish is also a great choice for protein. Beans (black beans, kidney beans, red beans, lentils, garbanzo beans) are a good source of protein, minerals, fiber and vitamins, and can be a protein substitute for meat.

Change is challenging, but so worth it. If you make a strong effort to improve your nutrition, your body will respond almost instantly. With habit and dedication, you will look and feel younger. Instead of feeling lethargic, you will feel an energy that will carry you through every day.

Simply giving up processed and sugary foods will make a difference that will amaze you. You will look and feel better from the inside out. And we promise you, it is worth it!

FEED YOUR BODY THE BEST FUEL YOU CAN

Make your calories count. Nutrient-dense calories fuel your body and keep you energized. Therefore the cleaner you eat (and more plant-based) the better you will feel.

Fruits and vegetables contain powerful vitamins, minerals, antioxidants to prevent disease. If you want to have a body free of diseases such as cancer, obesity, diabetes, high blood pressure, etc., then eat to live—don't live to eat. You may have heard that you should avoid fruit because it's just sugar. But whole fruit (not fruit juice) is loaded with nutrients you need, as well as fiber. Berries and cherries are full of vitamins and antioxidants. Some great choices are blueberries, strawberries, blackberries, loganberries, and dark cherries. Citrus fruits, including oranges, grapefruit, lemons and limes, are full of vitamin C and antioxidants.

Roots, fruits and greens you can blend for anti-inflammatory nutrition include turmeric, ginger, beets, pineapple, celery and kale.

Hey, we heard you groan. Here's the thing about kale. Kale has become the butt of the joke in many nutrition conversations. In reality, it is one of the most nutritious and healing foods you can consume. Get creative with this nutrient-rich vegetable and watch it work its magic from the inside out! If you're not a fan of the curly, chewy kale, buy a tender baby kale or Tuscan variety.

Here are some other vegetables that will pack more nutrition into every meal: spinach, dark lettuce, arugula, asparagus, green beans, brussels sprouts, tomatoes, squash, mushrooms, celery, carrots, beets, cucumber, eggplant, bananas, kiwi, melons, apples, peaches, nectarines, coconut. There are so many more. You get the idea.

AGELESS FATS

You also need fats for optimal brain function, but make sure you avoid processed vegetable oils. The best choices for Ageless Now fats are avocado oil, olive oil, and coconut oil. You can also get beneficial oils from olives, walnuts, almonds, hazelnuts, cashews, pine nuts, pecans, pistachios, pumpkin seeds, sunflower seeds, and any nuts or seeds turned into butter (with no added oils).

Living an Ageless Now lifestyle is not about losing weight. It's about brain health and making the decision now to change your diet. Keep in mind, this is just a guideline of how to live an Ageless Now life. This does not mean that you can't go out and celebrate a special occasion or have a cheat day. Nor is this about extreme weight loss, although living the Ageless Now way will likely change your weight. This is about living longer and healthier with an abundance of energy.

Losing excess weight also takes a huge load off your joints, specifically the hips and knees. Imagine filling a backpack with ten to twenty or more pounds in it and carrying it all day. At the end of the day, your joints would be screaming. The difference, of course, is that a backpack is easily removable and your desire to lose weight takes longer. But you don't have to do this all at once. Taking off a pound per week will eventually leave you feeling lighter and with abundant energy.

Here are some steps you can take toward making an Ageless Now commitment for your body and skin:

- Choose to give up soda for water or sparkling water.
- Replace cookies with veggies.
- Prepare meals and take them with you.
- Take time to enjoy the taste of fruits and vegetables.
- Learn to chew your food.
- Drink plenty of water.

- Throw out the junk food and replace it with healthy snacks.
- Give up processed sugar and eat fruit if you need something sweet.
- Shop for your favorite fruits and vegetables.
- Read about and research the foods you choose.
- Have a desire to be healthy that outweighs the desire to consume unhealthy food.
- Have a desire for energy and movement that outweighs the desire to sit.
- Make an appointment with your doctor to see check your bloodwork and see what nutrients you may be missing.

AGELESS SUPPLEMENTS

In case you missed that last bullet point, we'll say it again: Before you make any changes, it's imperative to have your doctor do a full blood workup to see what you are missing in your diet and what nutrients you are lacking. Unfortunately, many of our foods are lack the necessary nutrients, so taking extra in the form of supplements often does not hurt. We advocate for being safe and getting as much information as you can.

Here are some good supplements that work well for most:

Vitamin C, E. These are the basic powerhouse Ageless Now vitamins. Vitamin E works together with vitamin C, and is one of the most important antioxidants for the skin. It protects cell membranes from free radical damage. And since it's free radical damage that causes us to age, this combo is essential!

Vitamin D is necessary for building and maintaining healthy bones. That's because calcium, the primary component of bone, can only be absorbed by your body when vitamin D is present. Your body makes vitamin D when direct sunlight converts a chemical in your skin. (No, this doesn't mean you should skip the sunscreen.)

Turmeric helps as an anti-inflammatory and protects your joints. This vitamin is a powerhouse, and will definitely decrease joint pain. It also will help in muscle soreness recovery.

Ginger is a good anti-inflammatory for the joints and helps promote natural energy. Try a ginger tea for a natural boost.

Fish "krill" oil is necessary for brain function And this source of omega 3 fatty acids will not only keep your skin soft and supple, but will help prevent heart disease and also lower LDL cholesterol.

Calcium is necessary to keep your bones strong, especially for women.

Collagen promotes healthier skin and helps build the body's collagen that decreases as we age.

Milk thistle promotes healthier skin and free radicals, and helps your liver make the powerful antioxidants needed to generate skin cells. This can also make your complexion glow.

Chromium picolinate decreases sugar cravings (sugar in itself promotes faster aging), and high blood sugar levels are a BIG factor in the aging process. This is why it's crucial to strip your diet of sugar and junk food.

Glucosamine helps protect your joints. It is a compound that can help reduce wrinkles, fine lines, and liver spots, and also helps keep the skin supple from the inside out. It does this by inducing your skin's production of collagen. And as we said earlier, high collagen levels keep the skin plump and youthful.

Resveratrol is a phenol containing an antioxidant that is mostly found in red wine, red grape skins, peanuts, and raspberries. It helps alleviate the inflammation that leads to the aging of the inside of the body AND wrinkly skin.

L-arginine is an amino acid that encourages the release of a growth hormone from the pituitary gland. These hormones help you burn fat and increase lean muscle mass. It also improves libido, which, by the way, also can help keep you ageless.

It takes discipline and courage to live Ageless Now. We are bombarded with commercials that promote drug use when instead, food and movement are your better medicine—not pharmaceuticals. Take one day at a time. Small steps will yield big results.

SLEEP TO STAY AGELESS

Your body and your brain need sleep now more than ever. With sleep, your body repairs both physically and emotionally. When you have a wonderful night's rest you awake feeling as though you can conquer the world. But when you have a poor night's sleep, the next day can be quite a struggle. We all have bad nights, whether it's induced by hormones, alcohol, or emotions. You can get away with one night of sleep deprivation, but when it becomes frequent, the consequences are going to age you.

Sleep deprivation is a serious challenge, especially with hormonal changes primarily in women (not to say that men don't have sleep issues). There are multiple research studies on sleep deprivation that explain why it is crucial to get at least eight hours of sleep every night. Not only does a lack of sleep age you physically, you may feel it emotionally as well.

Lack of sleep can cause:

- Brain fog—inability to think clearly and make decisions.
- Inability to exercise.
- An increase in cortisol, which will end up as extra weight around the mid-section.
- Looking tired.
- Weight gain or loss.
- Lack of energy and less desire to exercise.
- Wrinkles.

SOLUTIONS TO IMPROVE YOUR SLEEP

- Don't drink caffeine after 1 p.m.
- Don't drink alcohol before bedtime.
- Exercise—go for a walk after dinner.
- Take a warm bath with lavender.
- Make sure your bed is comfortable and right for you.
- Meditate and practice deep breathing.
- Don't watch TV (especially the news) before bed.
- Don't take work to bed—leave it for the morning.
- Try to go to bed and wake up at the same time every day.
- Talk to a doctor about hormone replacement therapy.

You can't go back and change the beginning but you can start where you are and change the ending.

C.S. Lewis

4
MOVEMENT TO STAY FLEXIBLE AND FIT

You can't get beyond the body unless you free the body itself.

Ida Rolfe

Movement: No Grunting Required

Exercising to keep moving should not require superhuman effort. Have you ever gotten discouraged from working out? Or started a walking, biking, or class aerobics routine that you initially love but get discouraged because the movements are too difficult? Moving should be sustainable, and it will keep you younger longer than about any other practice.

We move constantly and it often is the unexpected twist or reach that can get us into trouble. Our goal is simple: Create a conscious movement or task for a subconscious result. When you train the body in specific patterns and movements it is better prepared for other activities—from walking to improving your golf game.

The I Am Ageless Now movements were developed specifically to provide a safe and reliable workout. This program is designed to help you expand the awareness of your body, both physically and emotionally. It will also help you increase flexibility and blood flow, focus on lengthening your muscles, activate your breath, and combine mantras as you move for greater peace of mind as you move.

GRAVITY AND THE INFLUENCE ON THE BODY

You know gravity is what keeps you grounded to the earth. But you may not have thought about how the earth's gravitational pull exerts constant pressure on the body, whether you're standing, sitting, or even lying down. The pressure challenges the body's core stabilizers and increases as the body progresses from lying down to sitting to standing. When your skeletal muscle system is strong, it helps you become more stable against any negative pressures of gravity, including any resistance from aerobic fitness movements.

IDENTIFYING APPROPRIATE PAIN-FREE RANGE OF MOTION

Range of motion refers to an individual's flexibility and mobility around a joint. As such, the initial range of motion describes the place where you can begin an exercise/movement while remaining pain-free.

The initial range of motion may be demonstrated by someone with an injury, and that is as far as they can flex a joint without feeling pain. The mid range of motion is a slightly larger than the initial range depending on the ability and mechanics. The end range of

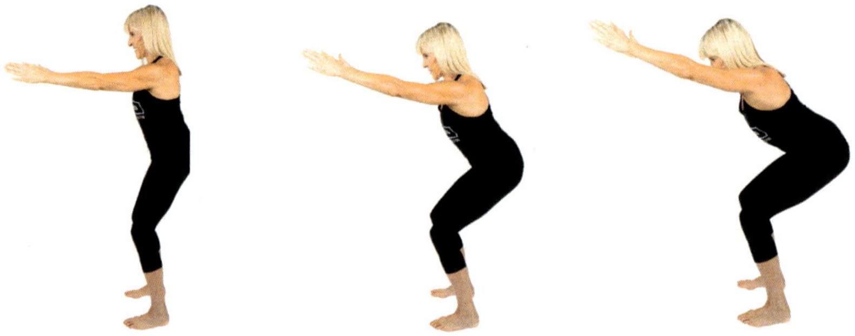

Initial Mid End

motion is the furthest point within the full range that one can move pain-free for their ability and in proper alignment.

As you become more familiar with the movements that will help you maintain your flexibility and function, you'll see the I Am Ageless Now exercise program includes those meant to target muscular imbalances, posture difficulties, and more, meant to help you increase your range of motion. If you have trouble rotating your head to look right or left in traffic, for example, some of these exercises are specifically designed to help you increase the rotation of those muscles. Others will help with balance and flexibility.

SETTING YOUR INTENTION

We talked earlier about the importance of mindset for Ageless Now living. It's also important when you're doing the movements to keep your mindset strong and positive. Movement may be new for you, and that's OK. You may have been inactive for a number of years, and that's OK too. It's not too late. Start where you are.

When you begin each movement, make sure to take a full breath in through the nose and exhale through the mouth completely. When you take these deep breaths, you will find it will help to decrease the sensitivity of certain areas that are more tender, such as the thighs. If you focus on your breath, you will find that you can work on an area longer and it becomes less sensitive. And, when you intentionally breathe through the exercise, you can move more fluidly with ease and enjoyment, positivity and energy.

Try and do both sides of your body equally because we have a tendency to favor one side over the other, especially when it comes to strength or balance. It's a good challenge to work on the weaker side equally to create symmetry and better balance of your body. As you do this, you will notice a change in better mobility and it's likely you'll feel less pain.

CONSCIOUS AND SUBCONSCIOUS MOVEMENTS

Conscious movements are those you perform with purposeful awareness. When you're first beginning these movements, it's good to be aware of each detail of the exercise, especially paying attention to how it feels in each section of the movement and how your body finds balance.

Subconscious movements are the things you do without being aware that you're doing them. One example is how you sit when you're driving your car, or how you simply walk, run, or how you perform any movement where you don't necessarily consciously think about how to do it. It's a pattern your body does simply without consciously working out how to do it.

It's important to train to be fit at both a conscious and subconscious level. If you dedicate a bit of time each day to consciously practice these movements, your conscious movements can eventually become subconscious. When this happens, you can focus on enhancing your new skills within each movement, which could include progressing into more complex versions of the movements.

Any movement, in any joint, has an effect on every other one of your joints up and down the body. This is known as the kinetic chain. When you have any injuries, even micro-trauma or strains in the muscles, joints, ligaments, and fascia in one area of the body, it can lead to pain and potentially postural or other issues in another area of the body along the kinetic chain.

When someone moves their head left or right, for example, a slight, almost imperceptible movement from the foot up through the kinetic chain allows this to occur. The action of turning the head creates small movements in the ankle without causing pain.

THE AGELESS BODY WORKOUT

Having access to the right equipment for these movements is important. This program doesn't require a lot—you can do most of these movements using equipment you may already have. A couple of things you may not have are a small ball (we use the Bender Ball, which Leslee developed several years ago), Gliding discs, tubing with handles, and the Rollga roller. You can use a different foam roller if you prefer. The Bender Ball and Gliding discs are available on our website, iamagelessnow.com. You will use a yoga mat for most of the movements as well, and you will also want to have a tennis ball and some tubing with handles.

The **Bender Ball** is a small exercise ball you'll use for a variety of movements. It's particularly useful to prop behind your lower back to ensure you don't injure your back. When you're placing the ball for each exercise, wedging the ball behind the low back is the best placement. You never want to extend so far that the low back is compromised in any way you shouldn't be feeling pain.

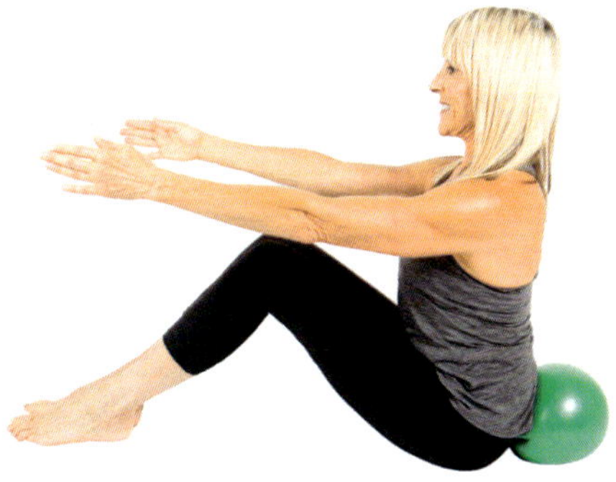

Make sure the ball is not too full. If it is, it will be very uncomfortable when you're performing exercises on the low back. On the other hand, an under-inflated ball won't give your back the support it needs. A happy medium is a full, soft ball that is a little squishy, and will protect the back during exercises.

The **Gliding Discs** are meant to be placed under your feet during exercise so you can do smooth graceful movements that firm, tone, and sculpt long, lean muscles. There is one set of discs that will slide easily on carpeting, and a different set for hard floors, depending upon where you exercise most. If you don't have or can't find Gliding discs, you can use paper plates, which slide on most surfaces. Make sure that you have the center of the foot on the disc and become used to it first before proceeding with the full range of motion. The Gliding discs can also be used under the hands when doing floor work focusing on the core and upper body.

When used correctly, Gliding discs can make an exercise easier for beginners, and for the more advanced, they can provide more range of motion and intensity to an exercise to strengthen and lengthen all major muscle groups of the body. For those using the Gliding discs for the first time, it is always better to introduce exercises that are slower and will help you get used to the gliding motion and establish your balance.

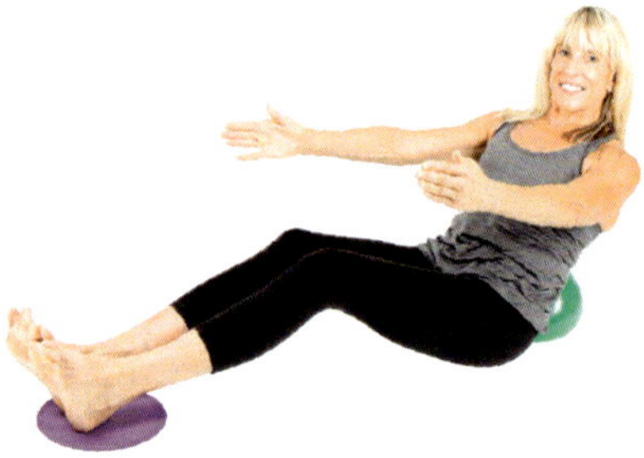

One of our favorite rollers is a **Rollga foam roller**. It has three contours: a narrow middle contour and two outer ridges specifically for the muscles and fascia to float through, which is beneficial to increase flexibility, blood flow and hydration to the tissue. When you begin rolling, make sure you begin gently, flossing the tissue. Add pressure (compression) and hold as directed in the movements.

Foam rolling is essential for staying ageless. Rolling the fascia helps diminish aches, pain and stiffness, and will increase your flexibility, hydration, blood flow, and range of motion. If you feel any pain while you're rolling, make sure you stop and assess the source of the pain. If the pain is intense, it's always best to check with your doctor before continuing.

There are many brands and types of rollers. If you are more sensitive a soft roller is better. And if you like deeper pressure try a harder or a denser one. The Rollga pictured here has three contours (middle one being narrower) and two ridges specifically for the muscles and fascia to float through, which is beneficial to increase flexibility, blood flow, and hydration to the tissue.

We use these tools specifically to help break apart inflamed fascia. This simple equipment also offers a surprising amount of support and can act as an extension of your body to create more stability and range of motion.

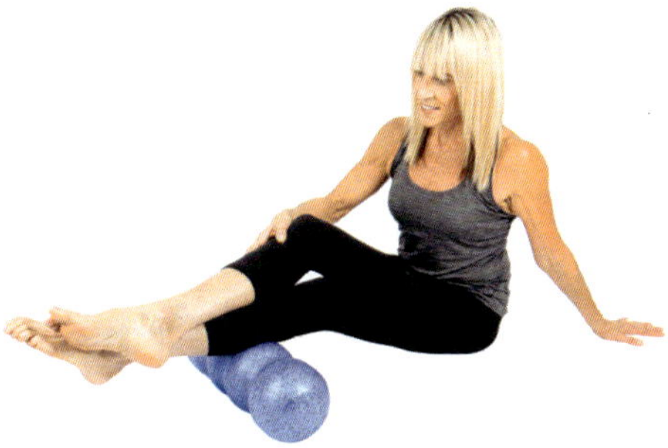

Here's what I know: I'm a better person at fifty than I was at forty-eight, and better at fifty-two than I was at fifty. I'm calmer, easier to live with. All this stuff is in my soul forever. Just don't get lazy. Work at your relationships all the time. Take care of friendships. Hold people you love close to you. Take advantage of birthdays to celebrate fiercely. It's the worrying, not the years themselves, that will make you less of a woman.

Patti LaBelle

If movement and activity is new to you, or you're just getting back to it after an injury or illness, please take the time to visit your physician and make sure these movements are right for you. They are designed to be gentle movements (as opposed to the boot camp workouts you may see online). We strongly discourage anyone from jumping into an aggressive training program when you haven't taken the time to assess your capability. You can progress with these movements to a point where you can do more aggressive movements, but start simple and listen to your body. We are certain that if you commit a few minutes EVERY day to some of these movements, you will begin to feel stronger, more flexible, and begin your journey to living the Ageless Now way.

The more functionally flexible you are the better your body will perform. This does not mean staying in a painful stretch for an extended period of time; it's more about what will align your body for success in other activities.

Each of the movements is outlined in the pages that follow, along with photos that show you the correct positioning. At the end of this section you'll find a few pages with recommended combinations that will give you a variety of daily routines you can combine for a great daily workout. As we mentioned before, this is not intended to replace physical therapy or medical advice; those you still need to get from a licensed medical professional.

The movements should be done on each side of the body and to your ability. Make sure to take the time to feel it in your body. Notice specifically where you feel a change in mobility, flexibility, less pain, etc. A section titled "Begin" will give you the details on how to perform each movement. The "Purpose" section of the exercise will describe the benefit to your body.

MOVEMENT 1

FOOT MASSAGE

You'd be surprised how much tension you hold in your feet. The feet have receptors that relate to many other organs in your body. Releasing tension in certain areas of your feet will positively affect other areas of your body. The feet have 20 muscles that give the foot its shape by holding the bones in position while they also expand and contract for movement. Massaging the feet while pressing on a tennis ball or roller will relax your feet, hydrate your fascia, and give you flexibility and energy for the rest of the movements.

WHAT YOU NEED: A tennis ball

BEGIN: Place a tennis ball on the ground directly underneath your toes with your heel on the ground. Flex and extend your toes around the ball while adding a bit of pressure. Do this approximately ten times, working the ball in between your toes. Next place the arch of your foot on the ball as though it were a bug and press down gently ten times. Press and release and do not forget to breathe through each pressing compression. Finally you will begin with the heel of your foot on the ball and rub back and forth from the back of your foot to your toes. Repeat the entire movement on the other foot. You can do this movement while sitting in a chair, while working, while you're brushing your teeth, or while you're standing in the kitchen making a meal.

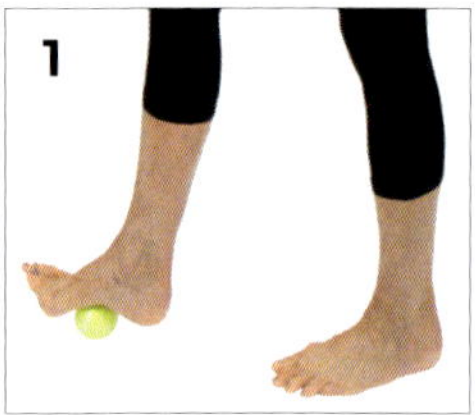

PURPOSE: Rolling the foot on the ball feels good and helps loosen the fascia of the foot. Your feet become sensitive for many reasons, but most often due to wearing inappropriate shoes, standing for long periods, or if you have plantar fasciitis.

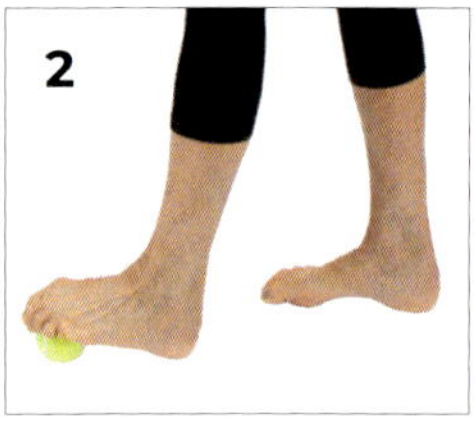

MOVEMENT 2

CALF MASSAGE

Massaging your calves will increase your ability to walk or run and improve balance and flexibility. This exercise will also help the function or your ankles, knees and hips.

WHAT YOU NEED: A tennis ball

BEGIN: Start seated on your mat and place the tennis ball under the middle of your right calf. Place your hands behind you. Next lean a bit forward to create pressure on the calf. Remember to breathe. Flex and extend your ankle ten times. Next you can cross your left thigh over the right, which will add weight and intensity to the calf. You can also move the calf side to side with your hands for more of a massage. Repeat on the other calf.

PURPOSE: This movement will stimulate the fascia of the calves. This area can be sensitive due to wearing high-heeled shoes, over-working your toes, or not stretching the calves enough. Calves are one area of the body that get extremely tight, so it is very important to do this movement frequently.

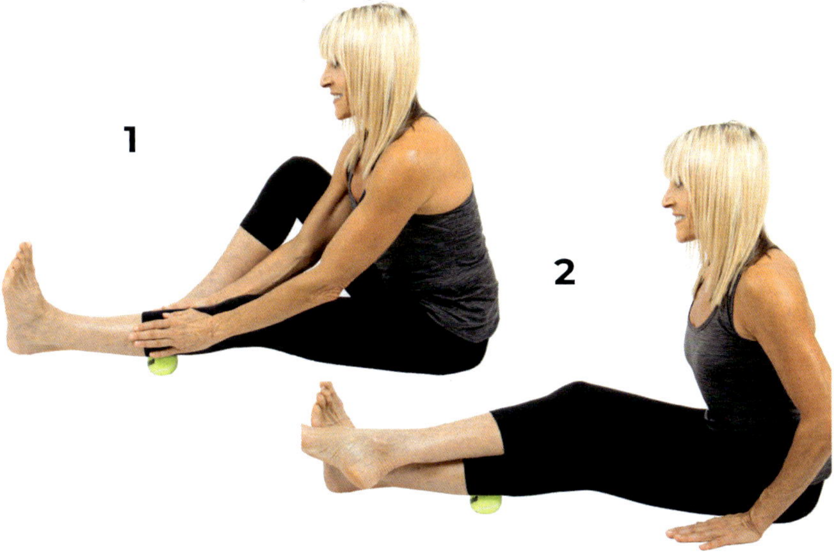

MOVEMENT 3

OUTER THIGH MASSAGE

This will help you to have more functional and flexible legs, especially if you're active in sports or other activities. It also feels great to massage the outer thigh before and after any workout.

WHAT YOU NEED: A tennis ball

BEGIN: Begin seated on your mat and place the tennis ball under the outer part of the right thigh. Place your left hand directly on the inner the left thigh and add gentle pressure just above the tennis ball ten times. You can hold for a few seconds and making sure to breathe through each pressing motion. Repeat on the left thigh.

PURPOSE: To massage the outer part of the thigh by stimulating the fascia in that region. This is a great exercise for the active runner or cyclist. This area can become sensitive due to wearing improper shoes, tight hamstrings, tight glutes, and activities such as running and cycling will contribute.

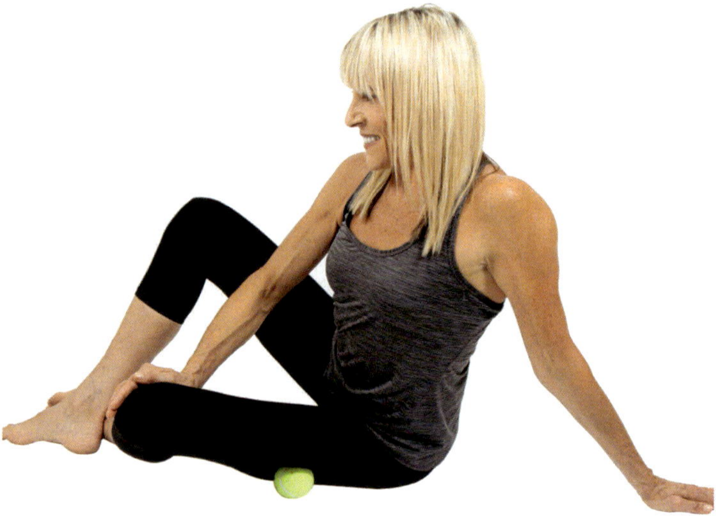

MOVEMENT 4

GLUTE MASSAGE

This is an essential massage for pain in the back and hips due to sitting. This will stimulate the area of the glutes that will give you better alignment of the rest of the body; this massage can even be done while sitting in a chair. It will be a bit painful at first, but the more you do this, it will start to feel better.

WHAT YOU NEED: A tennis ball

BEGIN: Begin seated on the mat and place the tennis ball directly under the right glute. Hands will be to the side of the body and slightly behind you to keep your body upright. Slowly let your knees sway or fall to the right as you feel the pressure on the ball, and return to the starting position. This is a sensitive area so only add as much body weight as is tolerable. For more of a massage you can lift the hips and make small circles on the ball, which gets very deep into the muscle tissue. Remember to breathe through the movement. For less body weight you can lie on your back or sit in a chair, placing the ball under the gluteus region and do the same movements as sitting. Repeat the movement on the left side.

PURPOSE: This exercise will massage and stimulate the fascia of the glutes. This area is particularly sensitive due to excessive sitting, sciatica, or weakness. This movement will help with doing squats and other exercises more efficiently.

1

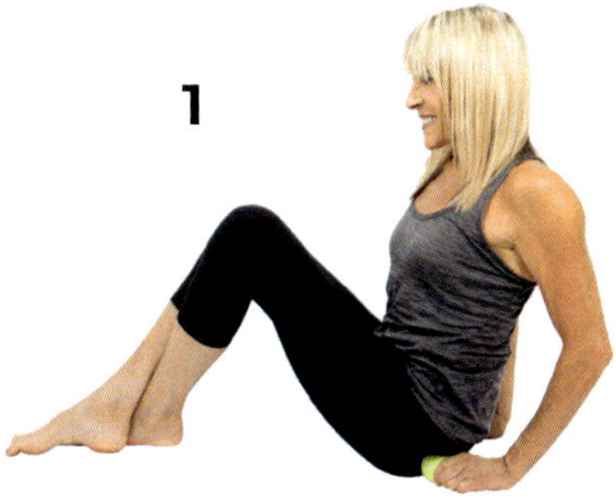

2

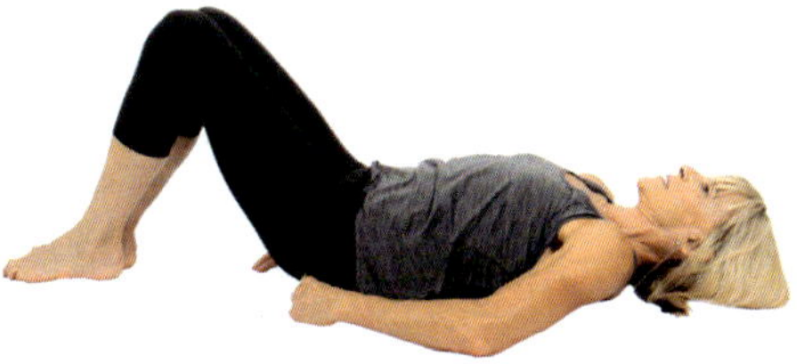

MOVEMENT 5

HIP FLEXOR MASSAGE

This is a wonderful massage for anyone who is active and or sits during the day, which shortens the hip flexors. This will restore the body back to balance and symmetry. Hip flexors become short from sitting, wearing high heel shoes and improper core training, leading to pain and dysfunction. When combined with the stretching techniques, you will have balance in the body.

WHAT YOU NEED: A tennis ball

BEGIN: Begin on your forearms lying face down and place the tennis ball in between the hip and thigh area of soft tissue. (This is a very sensitive area and placement for men is especially important.) Apply your body weight on the ball and take deep breaths. Stay in the position and rock gently side to side ten times. Repeat on the other side.

PURPOSE: To release the area of the front of the hip. When not addressed, this area will create issues in the low back, knees and hips, which can lead to greater problems.

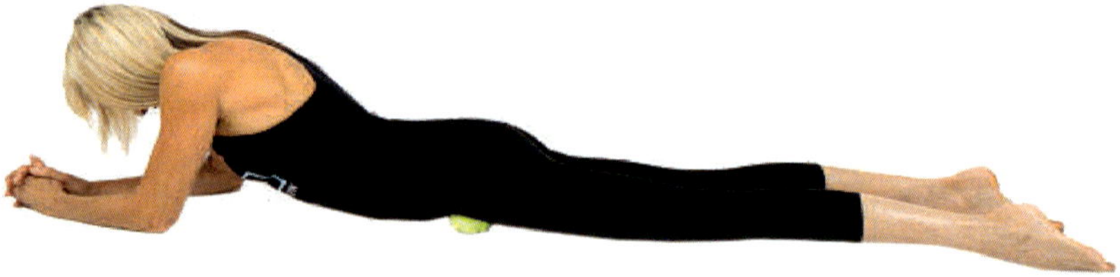

MOVEMENT 6

MASSAGE FOR YOUR QUADS (THIGHS)

This massage is an essential part of training because your quads are used for almost every movement—sitting up, sitting down, walking, running. You get the picture. Your quads can become tired and sore very easily, especially when they are overtrained.

WHAT YOU NEED: A tennis ball

BEGIN: Begin on the forearms on the mat, placing the ball directly in between your knee and your hip (right thigh). Next, apply your body weight directly on the ball. Slowly bend and flex the knee for more intensity and pressure while taking deep breaths. Inhale, straighten the knee, then exhale, bend. Move the ball to a different location (closer to the knee or thigh) and repeat ten times. The quads are a large complex area and need massage regularly. Repeat on the left thigh. You can also sit in a chair and place the ball in your right hand and massage the right thigh.

PURPOSE: To release the muscles and fascia of the thigh. When done regularly you will notice your thighs will have more vitality.

1

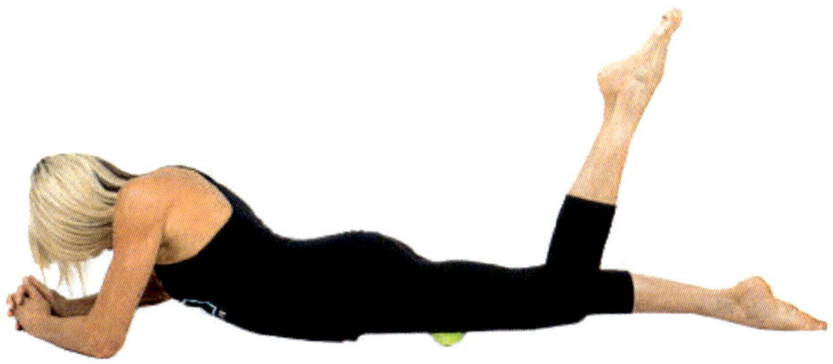

2

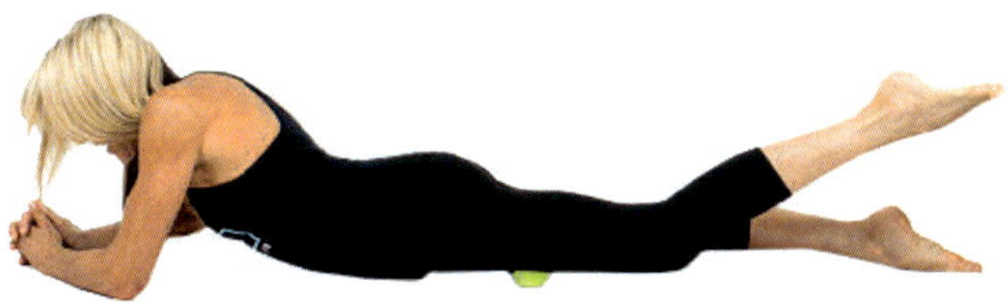

MOVEMENT 7

MASSAGE THE FRONT OF THE SHOULDERS

This massage is wonderful for anyone sitting at a desk for long periods of time and experiencing tight chest muscles and shoulders. This is also a great movement to do after a long drive.

WHAT YOU NEED: A tennis ball

BEGIN: Begin by holding the ball in your right hand and place the ball in between your left shoulder and chest. Gently press into the ball and massage, making small circles or just compressing into that area. Take deep breaths as you add pressure. Repeat on the right shoulder.

PURPOSE: The purpose is to release tight chest muscles (pectoralis) and the surrounding fascia. This area can become sensitive due to sitting over a computer, over-training the chest, sitting in a car, or sleeping only on one side.

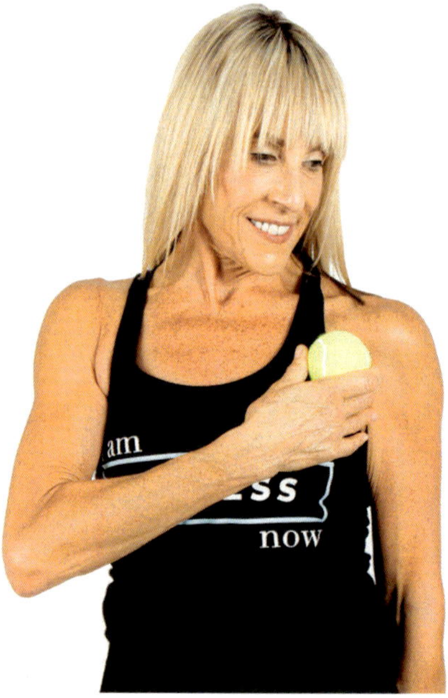

MOVEMENT 8

MASSAGE THE BACK OF YOUR SHOULDER

This is an essential massage for tension in the upper shoulder area of the back, which can be particularly sensitive due to long periods of sitting over a computer, driving, or poor posture.

WHAT YOU NEED: A tennis ball

BEGIN: Begin by either sitting in a chair, or against a wall or lying on your back on a mat (more intense version). Place the ball above the right shoulder blade and lean into it with your body weight. Take deep breaths and move the body a bit around the ball to find other areas that need compression around the shoulder.

PURPOSE: The purpose of this exercise is to release tension in the shoulder area as well as the muscles and fascia above the shoulder. We get very stiff from sitting over a computer, which can also lead to headaches.

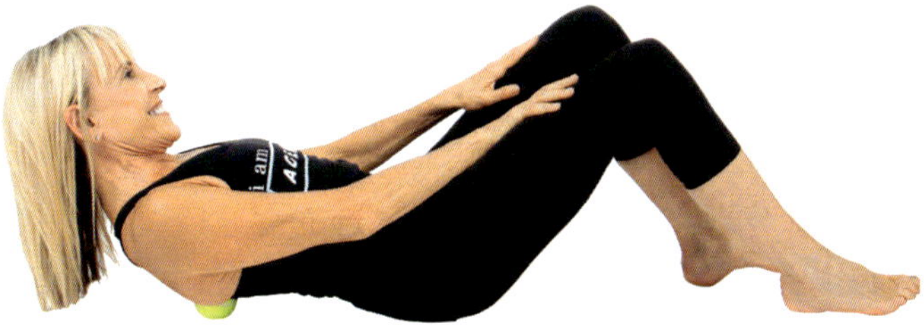

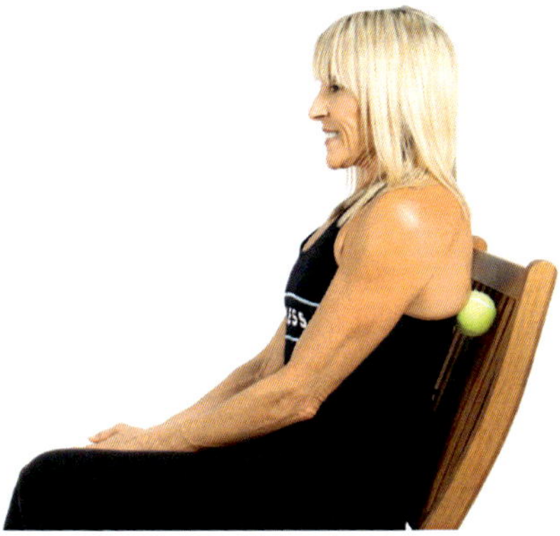

MOVEMENT 9

MASSAGE YOUR NECK

We so often hear, "My neck is so stiff!" This is an essential massage for anyone experiencing pain in the neck from sitting long periods of time over a computer or driving. This area is also very sensitive due to stress, incorrect core training, and habitual bad posture.

WHAT YOU NEED: A tennis ball

BEGIN: Begin by lying on your back and place the ball on one side of the neck. Gently turn the head in the same direction and hold the position taking deep breaths and try to relax. You can also place two tennis balls in a sock for each side of your neck.

PURPOSE: To release tension in the neck.

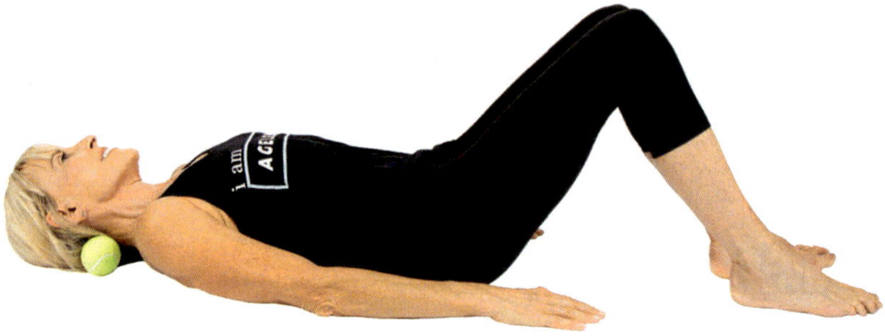

MOVEMENT 10

MASSAGE YOUR FOREARMS AND THIGHS

This is an easy to do exercise to massage both your forearms and legs. This is a quick fix for tired forearms and quads for anyone who sits during the day. Your forearms can be sensitive due to sitting at a computer, texting, carpal tunnel, over planking or push-ups.

WHAT YOU NEED: A tennis ball

BEGIN: Begin in a seated position. Place the ball on your right thigh. Start to roll the ball the length of your thigh with the palm of your hand. Next place the ball under the forearm and repeat rolling the length of the thigh ten times Add gentle pressure with the hand. Take nice deep breaths while doing so. Repeat on the other side.

PURPOSE: To release tension in the forearm and to massage the thigh.

1

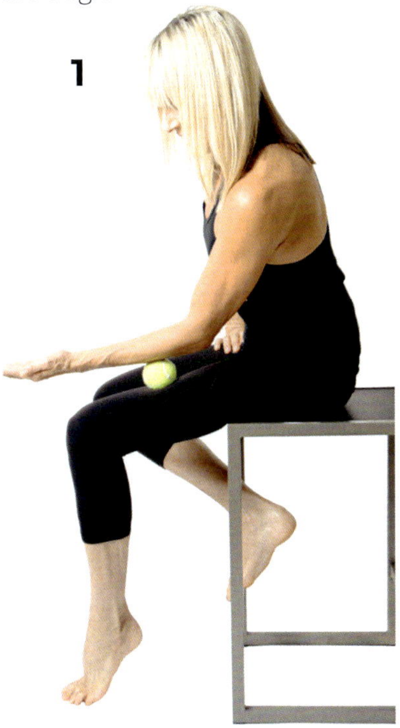

2

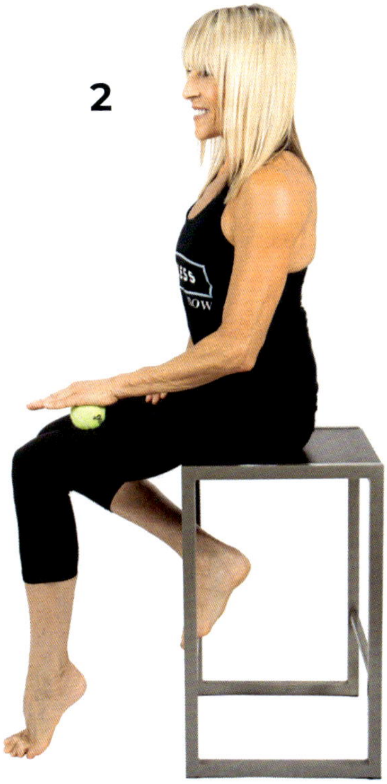

MOVEMENT 11

STRETCH YOUR CALVES

This is a great exercise to have more efficient functional calves that may be tight. If you love to walk or jog, you will want to do this beforehand, to stretch and lengthen the calves. The foot and ankle play a role in the function of the rest of the body. When doing this stretch, make sure to take deep breaths and keep good alignment for best results.

WHAT YOU NEED: Yoga mat

BEGIN: Begin by stepping back into a lunge position with your right foot starting from a hip-width position (or wider) for balance. Make sure all ten toes are facing forward. Next reach your arms in front of you, shoulders straight ahead. Start to bend your left knee slightly until you feel a stretch in the right calf.

You can feel in your own body if you want to bend the left knee more to create a bigger stretch in the right calf. Also make sure to keep your neutral spine and not flex forward as it will lessen the stretch. Repeat bending and straightening the left knee ten times and repeat on the other side. Make sure to breathe through the exercise to enhance flexibility.

PURPOSE: To lengthen and stretch the calves.

1

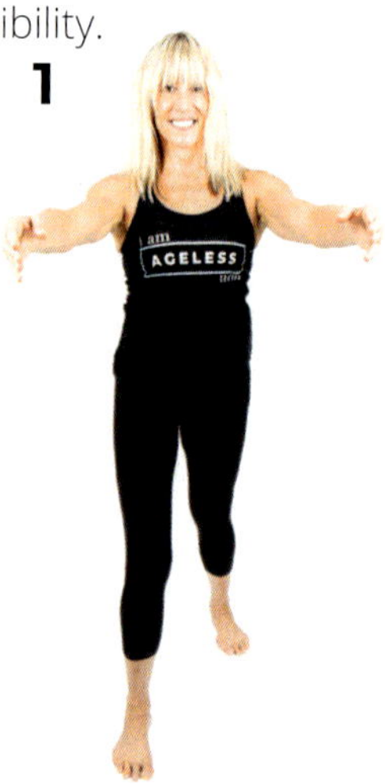

2

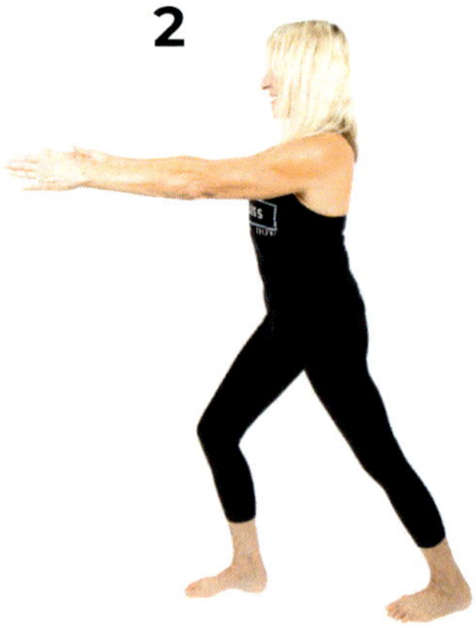

MOVEMENT 12

STRETCH THE FRONT OF YOUR HIPS

This is such an important exercise for everyone! Think about how much time people spend sitting and getting stiffer by the minute (and then wonder why they have back issues). When you do this movement a few times a day you will start to feel less back pain and more agility. Not only is this important for those who sit, but for golfers or tennis players this is a must. Your back and hips will have a new life!

WHAT YOU NEED: Yoga mat

BEGIN: Begin by stepping back in a lunge position with the right foot from a hip width or wider position and all ten toes facing forward. Same as the calf stretch. Next reach your arms above your shoulders until you feel the front of the right hip lengthen and stretch. Start to slightly bend the left knee while keeping your arms above you, and feel the stretch start to intensify. Think of reaching upward and not arching the back but keep neutral spine for efficiency. Make sure to breathe through the movement and, as always and take the time to feel it. Do this ten times and repeat on the other side.

PURPOSE: To lengthen the front of your hip for better function.

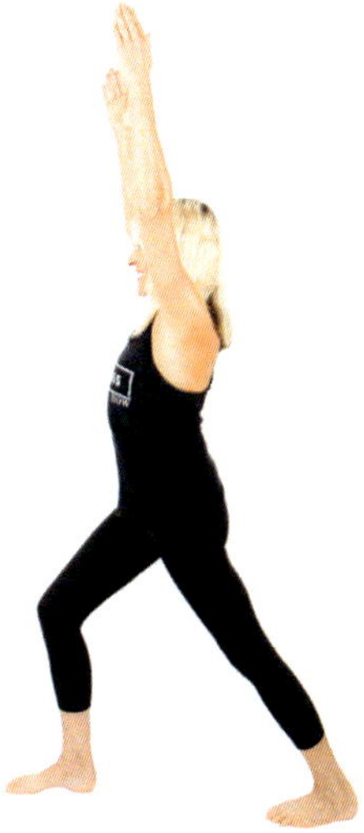

MOVEMENT 13

STRETCH THE BACK OF YOUR HIPS AND LEGS

This is such an essential exercise and stretch for the hamstrings and glutes for function. These muscles get especially tight with sitting log periods or from overtraining that can lead to back pain or injuries. When you do this you will feel the back of the leg lengthen and stretch for function. Once again, we spend so much time in dysfunctional positions that it affects the glutes and hamstrings, causing them to shorten and become weak. This exercise is also good to do before you go on a walk or run or even before playing tennis to give you more power and efficiency.

WHAT YOU NEED: Yoga mat

BEGIN: Begin by stepping back in a lunge position with the right foot from a hip width or wider position with all ten toes facing forward (same position as the front of the hip stretch). Next reach your arms in front of you then move slightly below the left knee as though you were picking up an object using your glutes and hamstrings, not your low back. Start to slightly bend the left knee and feel the stretch in the back of the left leg. Make sure once again to keep a neutral spine and engage your core here due to the position. Use your breath as you reach to enhance the stretch. Do this ten times and repeat on the other side of the body.

PURPOSE: To lengthen and strengthen the back of your hip.

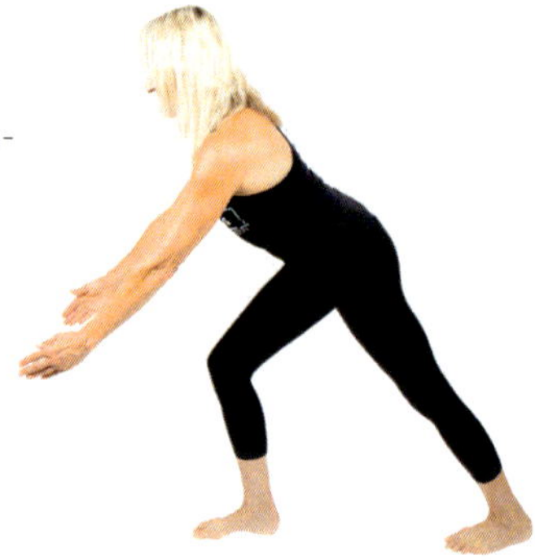

MOVEMENT 14

STRETCH THE SIDE OF YOUR HIPS

This is an essential exercise and stretch for anyone who plays rotational sports like golf or tennis, and it's also important for the function and mobility of the hips and back. Our hips can get sore and tight from many daily activities and this movement will help release and give them more mobility and stability. If you sit for long periods and then go to do an activity before warming up the hips, you will have issues. If you want to get one up on your golf or tennis pals make sure to do this daily!

WHAT YOU NEED: Yoga mat

BEGIN: Begin by stepping back in a lunge position with the right foot from a hip width or wider position and all ten toes facing forward (same position as the front of the hip stretch). Next reach your arms over your shoulders while keeping your neutral spine. Slowly start to side bend to the right, stretching away from the right hip as much as possible. Keep a slight bend in your left knee. Next reach to the left slowly. Repeat the movement side to side ten times and make sure to breathe to enhance flexibility. Repeat on the left.

PURPOSE: To lengthen the side of your hips and spine.

1 2

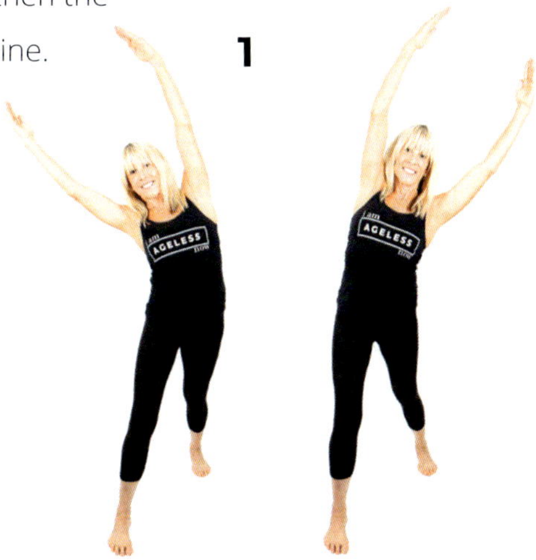

MOVEMENT 15

LENGTHEN AND STRETCH YOUR HIPS

Similar to lengthen and stretch the side of the hips, it is equally important to move them in all directions combined with moving the spine. Moving the hips and spine together helps for any rotational sport or activity and decreases the potential of back pain or injuries when you use your legs and hips rather than the back to pick up an object. When you combine this movement with the other hip movements, you will create very functionally strong hips.

WHAT YOU NEED: Yoga mat

BEGIN: Begin by stepping back in a lunge position with the right foot hip width or wider with all ten toes facing forward (same position as lengthening the front of the hips). Next, reach your right arm over your head and flex the spine to the right while reaching your left arm in front of your chest. Next, reach your left arm over your head and flex the spine to the left while reaching the right arm across the chest. The second part is to then reach your right arm below the left knee while rotating the spine and return to standing position. You can reach the left arm behind you for a greater stretch for the hips and upper back. Breathe through the rotation. Do this movement 10 times and repeat on the left.

PURPOSE: To lengthen the front and the back of the hips in more than one direction.

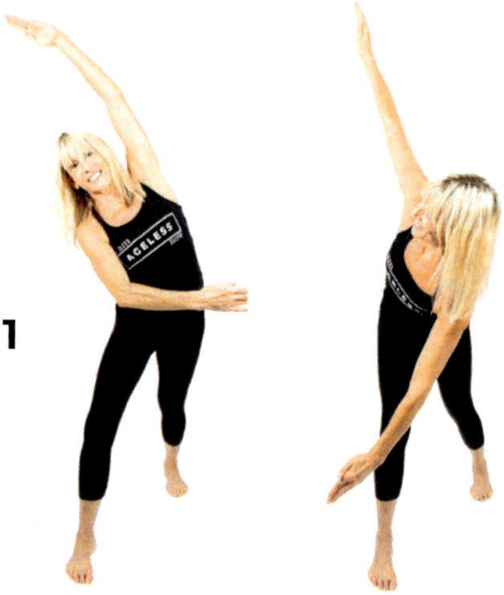

1 2

MOVEMENT 16

LUNGING WITH GLIDING DISC OR PAPER PLATE

This series ramps up the intensity of lunging without compromising your joints. You will still want to move at your range of motion and at your speed. This is so great for anyone looking to add a bit of cardio intensity or just increasing their flexibility. This series will also lengthen and strengthen the glutes for functional activities such as golf, tennis, etc. You will begin to find your glutes get stronger and more efficient by adding in this series of movements.

WHAT YOU NEED: Gliding disc or paper plate

BEGIN: Begin with the gliding disc under the right foot in an upright position. Next, slowly lunge back until you feel your left thigh engage. Reach your arms to shoulder height and return. Repeat 10 times on each side. Next, begin with the Gliding disc under the right foot in a hinged forward position and slowly lunge, reaching the hands below the left knee to engage the left hamstring and glute. Repeat 10 times on each side.

PURPOSE: To lengthen the glutes/hip flexors through full and half range of motion.

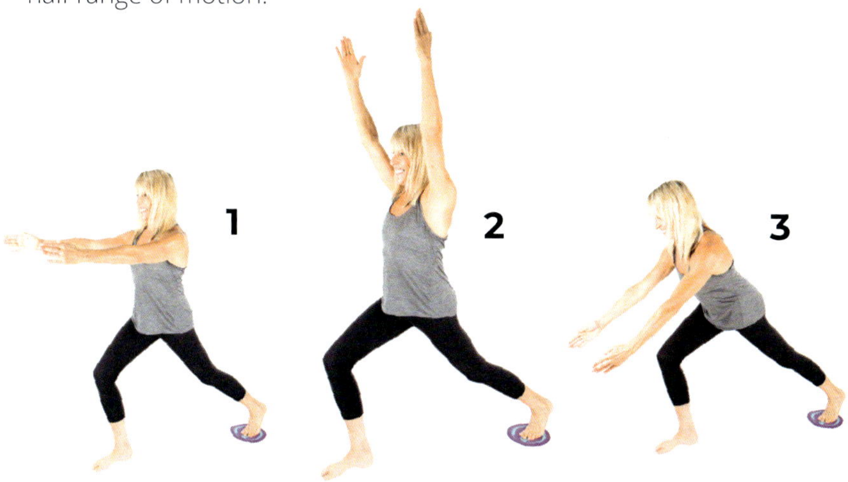

MOVEMENT 17

SKATER WITH GLIDING DISC OR PAPER PLATE

This is also a great series of movement exercises guaranteed to strengthen the glutes and hips for all functional activities. As mentioned previously, this will ramp up your cardio and keep your hips strong and flexible without impact or damaging the joints. Be sure to work at a range of motion and speed that is comfortable on both the knees and hips! You will gain power in all other activities.

WHAT YOU NEED: Gliding disc or paper plate

BEGIN: (1) Place the Gliding disc under the right foot. Next, take your right foot and slide it to the side and return with a straight knee while bending the left to activate the inner thighs. Repeat 10 times on each side.

(2) Next, place the Gliding under the right foot and slide outward, bending the left knee. Reach forward with the right hand to focus on the left hamstring and return. Repeat 10 times on each side. **(3)** Next place the Gliding under the right foot and slide outward, bending the left knee. Reach over the left knee and return to the starting position, as you will activate more of the side of the hip. Repeat 10 times on each side. **(4)** Next place the Gliding under the right foot and slide outward, bending the left knee. Place your hands behind your back, crossing your right leg behind as though you are skating to engage the glutes. Repeat 10 times on each side.

PURPOSE: To lengthen and strengthen the glutes, the side of the body, and the upper back.

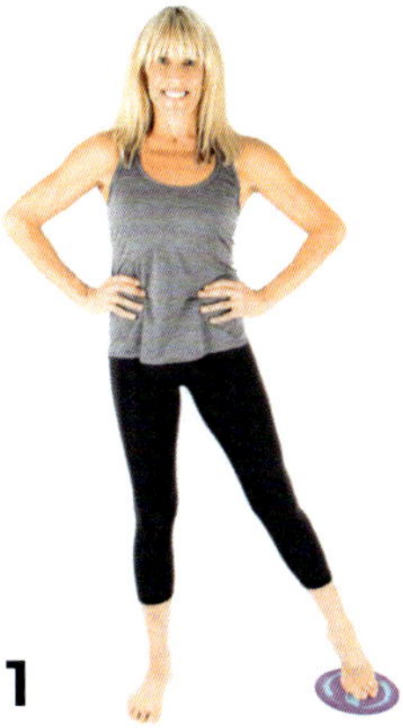

1

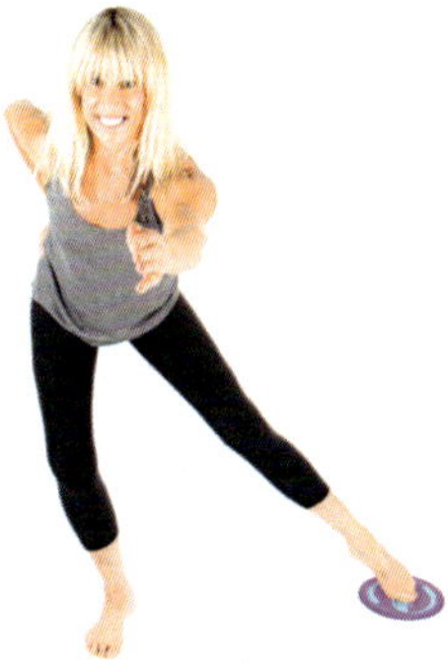

2

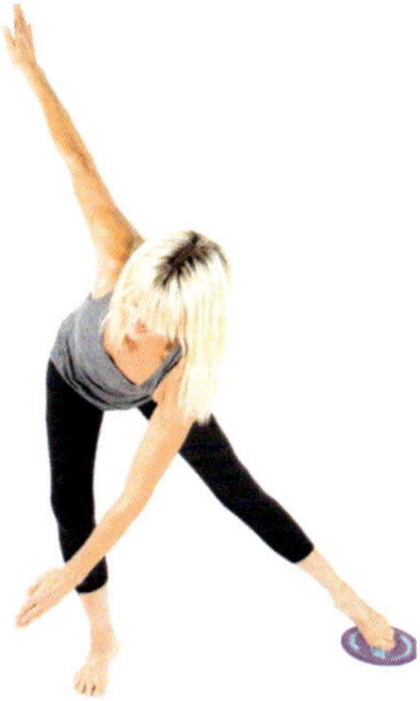

3

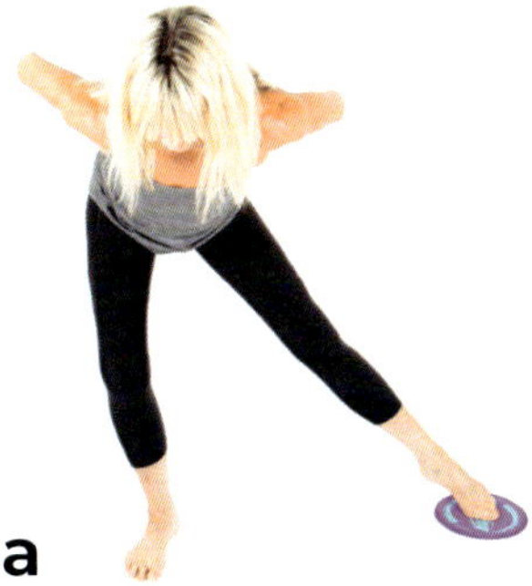

4a

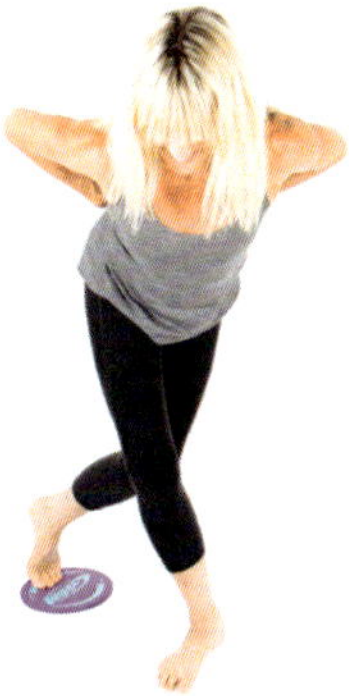

4b

MOVEMENT 18

PLANK WITH GLIDING DISC OR PAPER PLATE

This core exercise is guaranteed to strengthen the core, shoulders, and back for a strong and healthy body without impact on the joints. The core is crucial for all activities and the Gliding enhances the basic plank and takes it to a new level. Planking can always be done on a wall or chair without the use of discs or being on the floor if you have wrist issues. Keep in mind if you do fall you have to get up, and planking is a way to strengthen the body efficiently. If you have wrist issues then always use your forearms.

WHAT YOU NEED: Gliding disc or paper plate

BEGIN: Begin by placing the discs under all ten toes. Engage your core! Take a breath in and as you exhale pull the navel to the spine to protect the back. Next extend your knees and hips pushing the disc away. Return to the starting position and lower your knees if you need a break. If you have the strength, keep extending and bending the knees 10 times before you need a break.

PURPOSE: To strengthen the core while moving the extremities from the center of the body.

1

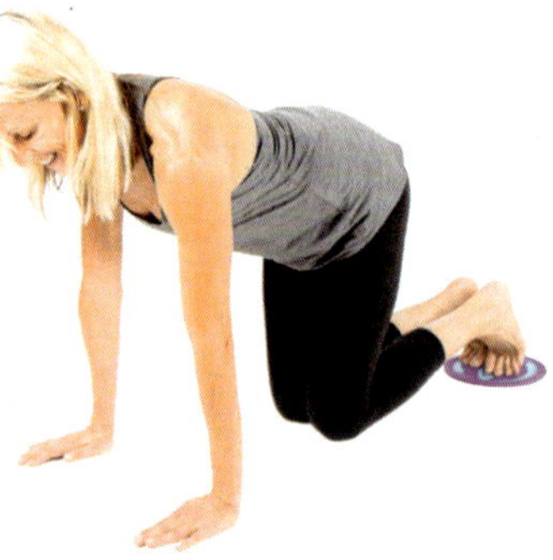

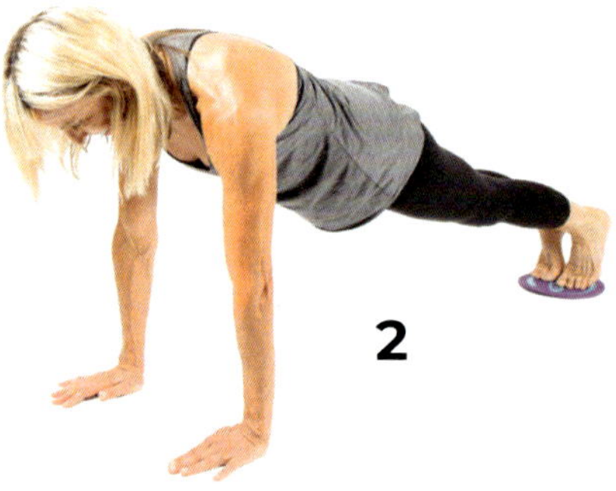

2

MOVEMENT 19

PLANK WITH GLIDING DISC VARIATIONS

This movement is more challenging as it requires more core strength, but it's good to move the body in more than one plank position for variety and function. This will challenge your core and bring up your heart rate, and make your body more functional and strong for other activities.

WHAT YOU NEED: Gliding disc or paper plate

BEGIN: Begin in the basic plank position either on the hands and knees or on the forearms with one disc or both discs under the feet.

Variations

(1) Leg to the Side: Begin in a plank position. Place one disc under the right foot and take the right leg out to the side and return, focusing on engaging the inner thighs and core. Repeat 10 times on each side.

(2) Mountain Climber: Begin in a plank position. Place one disc under the right foot. Next, bring the right knee to the left elbow, focusing on the obliques. Repeat 10 times on each side.

(3) Forearm Dolphin: Begin in a forearm plank position. Place both feet on the disc, maintaining the forearm plank. Next, lift the hips to a pike and return, focusing on the core. Repeat 10 times on each side.

PURPOSE: To strengthen the core while moving your extremities in different positions.

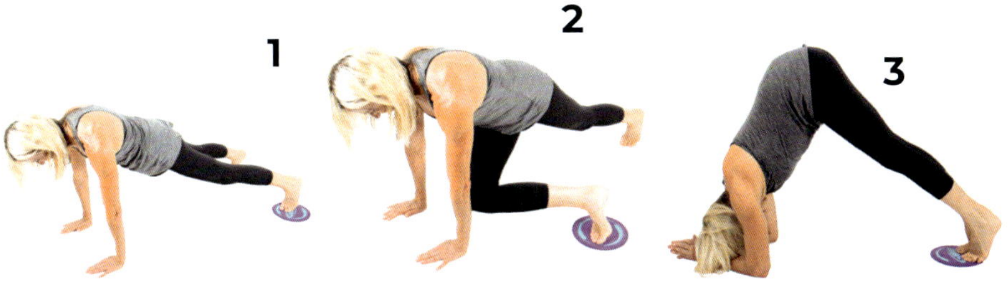

MOVEMENT 20

BENDER BALL SQUATS/STAGGERED/BALANCE

This series is great to strengthen the glutes, hamstrings and inner thighs for function and life! We need to get up and down all day, so why not be prepared? Your backside will be stronger and better looking for an ageless body. The ball is the best tool to align your hips and knees. Squatting when you hinge backward keeps you out of knee pain and is better for the back. You can always use a chair to hold onto if necessary, but if you can, work on balance and strength and find the range of motion that fits your body.

WHAT YOU NEED: Bender Ball

BEGIN: (1) Begin hip width apart; place the ball in between the thighs, above the knees. To activate the inner thighs, reach the arms forward for counterbalance. Next, place the weight in the heels and squat, sending the tailbone back, and return. Imagine sitting in a chair as you straighten your knees activate your inner thighs. Repeat 10 times on each side. **(2)** For variation place the right foot behind the left when you squat and focus on the right glute. It is slightly more intense but adds variety to your squat. **(3)** For the hardest version place one foot on the ball and slowly perform a one-leg squat.

PURPOSE: To lengthen and to strengthen the hips and inner thighs.

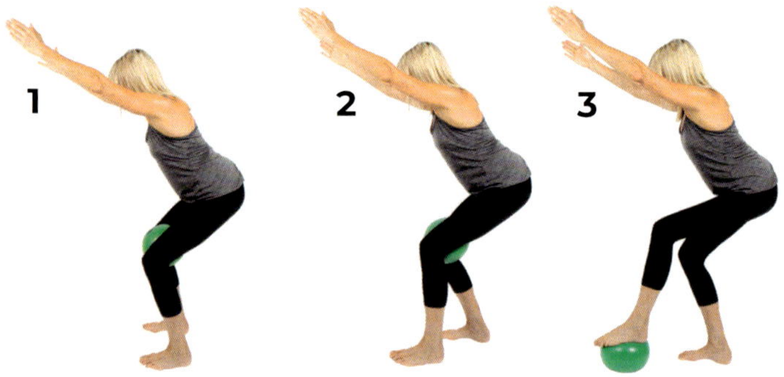

MOVEMENT 21

BENDER BALL SKATER BALANCE

We all need balance training as we age as it crucial for life, so why not practice in a functionally safe environment? You can always place your hand on a chair if necessary. This movement will strengthen the inner thighs, quads and glutes. This will keep you agelessly balanced. You can begin this movement without using the ball and get your alignment first, then add the ball for intensity. You will ultimately feel the supporting hip and thigh working to stabilize which is a good thing to strengthen.

WHAT YOU NEED: Bender Ball

BEGIN: Begin by placing the ball under the right foot to the side, but not weight bearing on the ball. Slowly squat with the left hip while putting very little pressure on the ball. Keep lowering and lifting while engaging the supporting side leg—it is like a side squat. Reach the arms in front of the body or reach across the left knee. Only move to the point that you can keep control. Repeat 10 times on each side.

PURPOSE: To create balance on the supporting leg while moving the other.

1

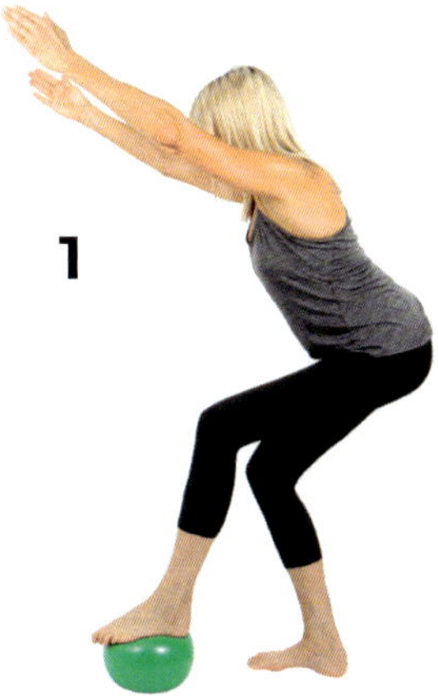

2

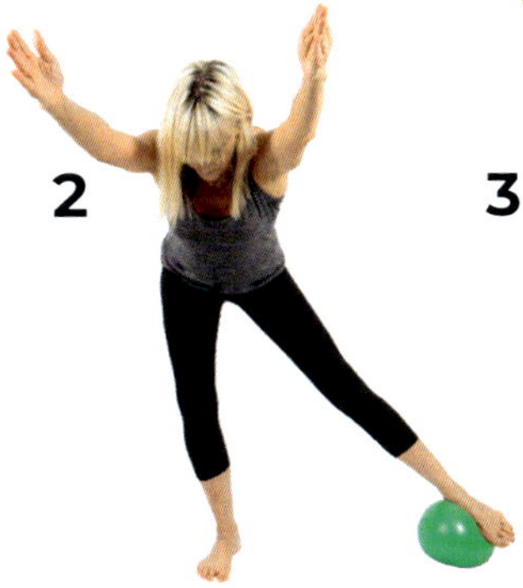

3

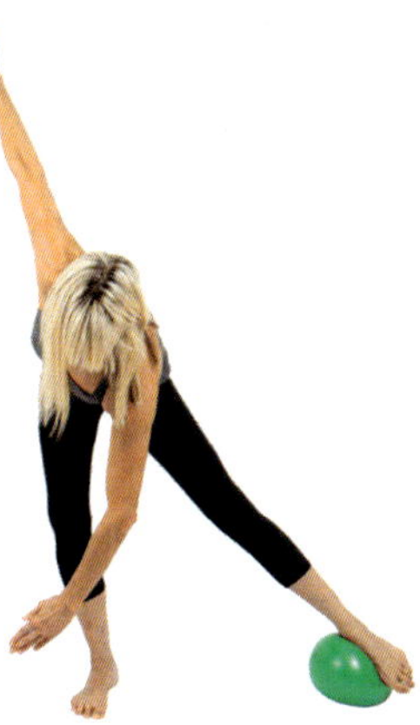

MOVEMENT 22

BENDER BALL SQUAT WITH BALANCE

This exercise will strengthen your glutes and inner thighs while adding a balance challenge for an ageless body! Balance training is so important to stay ageless and this exercise can be done providing great results. Make sure to work in your range of motion and hold onto a chair if you need assistance.

WHAT YOU NEED: Bender Ball

BEGIN: Begin with the ball in between the thighs above the knees next move into a squat while lifting the right foot off of the floor, focusing on balancing on the left. Keep the hips as neutral as possible. Repeat 10 times on each side.

PURPOSE: To lengthen and strengthen the working hip and glutes while focusing on balance.

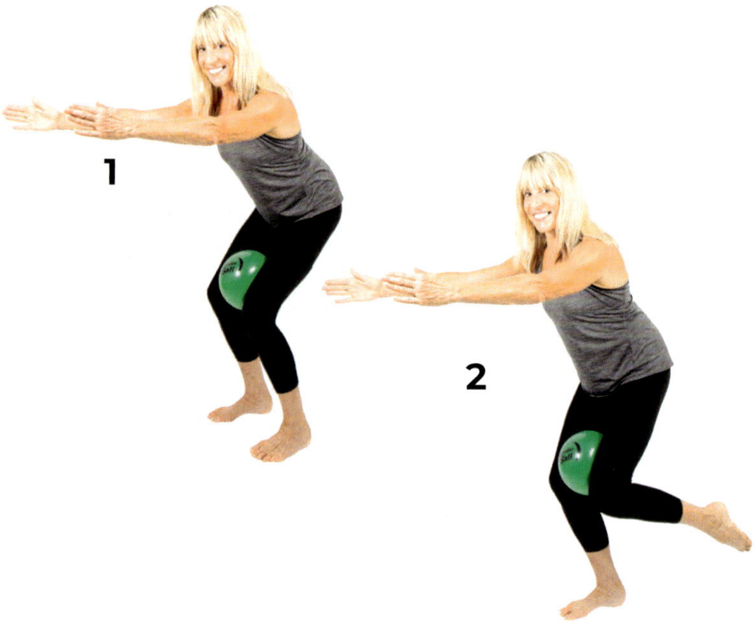

MOVEMENT 23

BENDER BALL DIRECTIONAL LUNGES WITH REACHES

This series of lunges mimics what we do in life, from picking up a box to putting it on a shelf. You will increase strength, flexibility and core for an Ageless Now body. If you do all of the variations, you'll find it's also cardio. Make sure to lunge back, finding your range of motion that's appropriate for your knees and back. Keep a neutral spine.

WHAT YOU NEED: Bender Ball

BEGIN: (1) Begin hip width apart and step back into a lunge with the right foot while reaching your arms shoulder height, return to starting position and alternate by lunging back on the left foot 10 times. **(2)** Begin hip width apart and step back in a lunge with the right foot reaching the arms over the shoulders, return to starting position and alternate by lunging back on the left foot 10 times. **(3)** Begin hip width apart and step back with the right foot reaching your hands below the left knee, return to starting position alternate by lunging back on the left foot 10 times. **(4)** Begin hip width apart and step back in a lunge with the right foot rotating your torso in the same direction, return to starting position alternate by lunging back foot on the left 10 times. **(5)** Begin hip width apart and step back in a lunge with the right foot reaching your arms over your shoulders and flexing your torso to the same side, return to starting position and alternate by lunging back on the left foot 10 times.

PURPOSE: To lengthen and strengthen the hips.

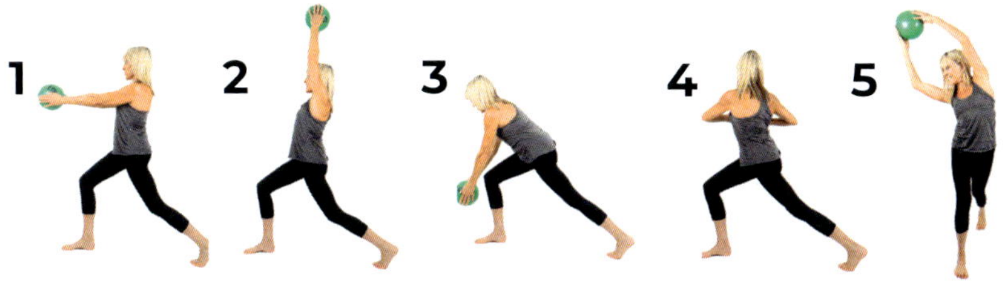

MOVEMENT 24

BENDER BALL LUNGES TO THE SIDE

This series mimics everyday activities in life or sports. Not only are you moving the entire body but you will be strengthening the core, legs, hips and upper body. Make sure to move where your body needs to go and never to push to where you feel knee or back pain. Keep your spine neutral and core engaged. Breathe through the movement to increase flexibility, mobility and focus! This will add a bit of cardio and give you a strong ageless body!

WHAT YOU NEED: Bender Ball

BEGIN: (1) Begin by lunging or stepping out to the right while flexing the right knee with your arms at shoulder height, rotate to the same side, return to starting position and alternate to the left 10 times, focusing on the core. **(2)** Begin by lunging or stepping out to the right while flexing the right knee and reach your arms below the right knee, return to starting position and alternate to the left 10 times, focusing on the right hamstring and glute. **(3)** Begin by lunging or stepping out to the right while flexing the right knee and reach your arms over your head while leaning to the right, return to starting position and alternate to the left 10 times, focusing on the core.

PURPOSE: To lengthen and strengthen the outer and inner muscles of the hip.

1

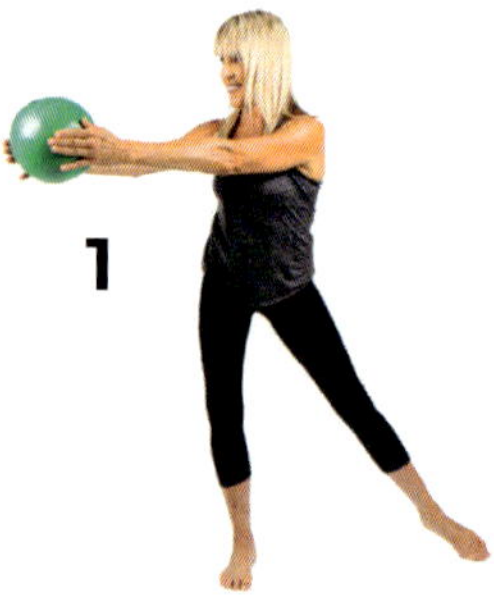

2

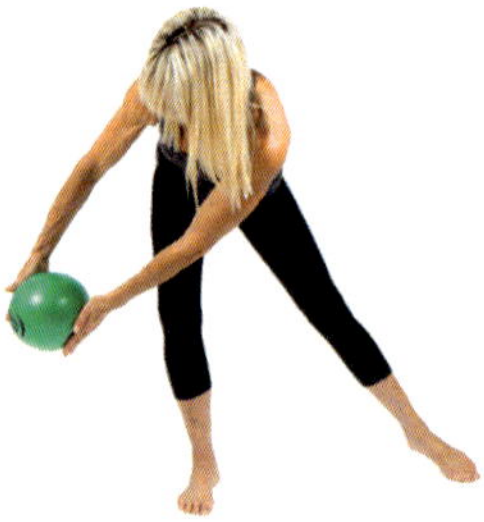

3

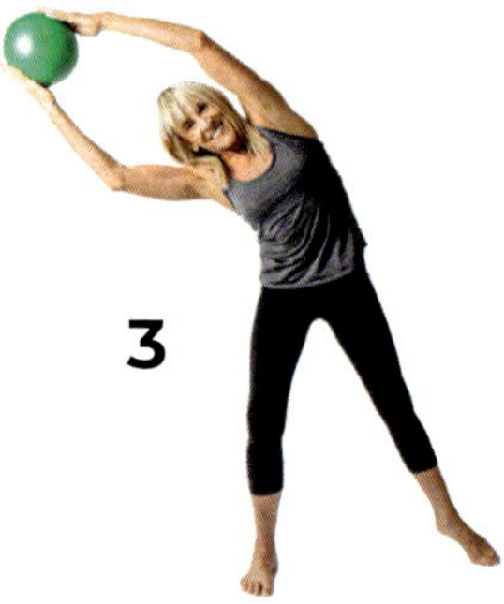

MOVEMENT 25

SEATED CORE WITH BENDER BALL

This series with strengthen the core without ever compromising the low back. The ball will protect your back by decreasing the use of your hip flexors for an ageless functional core! Don't be surprised when you feel the front of the body quiver. You are decreasing the use of the hip flexors and making the core do its job unlike any other exercise you may have done in the past! Do make sure to only move to that point and never too far back as you do not need to.

WHAT YOU NEED: Bender Ball, yoga mat

BEGIN: (1) Begin sitting on your mat, wedge the ball directly behind the low back/hip area (bunny tail). Make a small C curve with the low back while keeping your upper back straight. Hinge back until you feel the front of the body shake a bit. Next gaze upward with your eyes while your arms are directly in front of you. This is the initial starting position remember to breath through this section. **(2)** Begin in the same position alternate your arms over your shoulders 10 times. **(3)** Begin in the same position and reach both arms over your shoulders for more intensity 10 times. **(4)** Begin in the same position, lower your right elbow to the mat rotation your upper back next, return alternate to the left 10 times.

PURPOSE: Lengthen and strengthen the core.

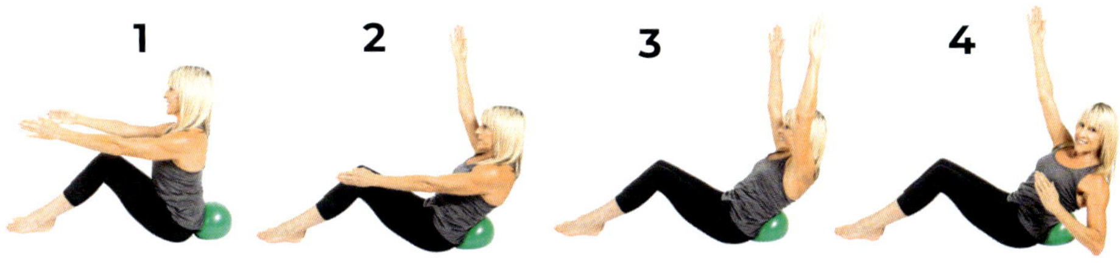

MOVEMENT 26

SIDE-LYING CORE WITH BENDER BALL

This series is the ultimate ageless waist whittler and core activator. You will strengthen the obliques for function and strength. It is very difficult to activate the obliques but not in this particular exercise, as you may find your core will quiver on this one as well! Unlike crunches this makes you utilize the body against gravity and work more efficiently for an extremely strengthened core.

WHAT YOU NEED: Bender Ball, yoga mat

BEGIN: Begin lying on the left side by placing the ball in between the ribs and the hips. Next, place the right hand on the floor and the left hand cradling your head. Initiate the movement first by activating the right side of the body. Next, lift your torso until you feel your core engage. Think of being in between two glass panels to help you lift straight up and down. For a more advanced move you can take your right hand off the floor. Repeat 10 times on each side.

PURPOSE: To lengthen and strengthen the obliques.

1

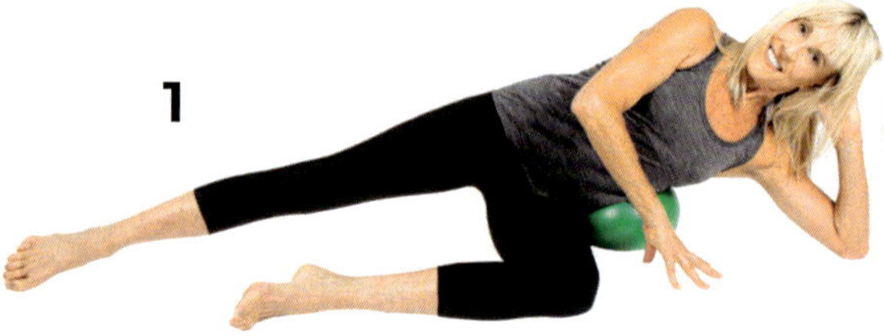

2

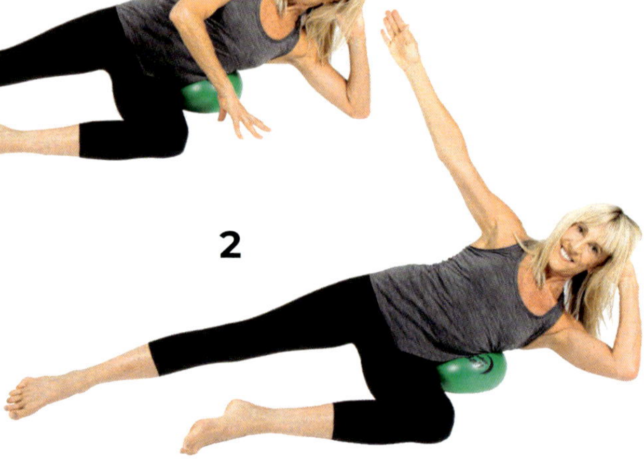

MOVEMENT 27

HANDS AND KNEES BALANCE WITH BENDER BALL

This exercise is improves core, shoulder strength and balance while on you hands and knees. As we age it is important to train the core in many positions for an ageless body. Also because your knees are on the ball it is more comfortable for anyone with knee issues. And, once again a planking core work is essential as we age if we should have to get up from the floor.

WHAT YOU NEED: Bender Ball, yoga mat

BEGIN: Begin on your hands and knees unless you have wrist issues—if you do, begin on your forearms. Next place both knees on the ball not fully weight bearing as you are on your toes. Remember to engage your core. Lift the right foot off the floor, return and alternate with the left.

PURPOSE: To activate the core.

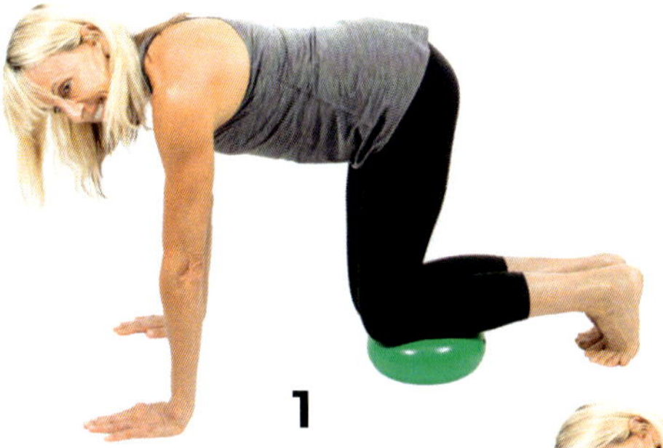

1

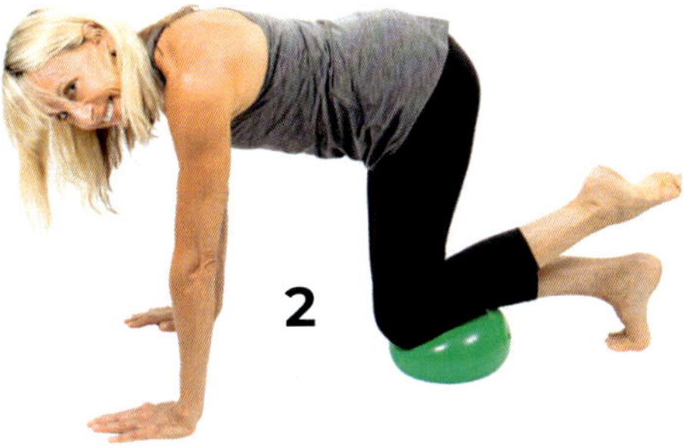

2

MOVEMENT 28

HAND BALANCE WITH BENDER BALL

This is another plank with a challenge of balance. By placing the hand on the ball you will want to engage the core even more. Think of a good strong neutral spine. Just by having your hand on an unstable surface is going to allow you to feel as though you are working harder and with more concentration.

WHAT YOU NEED: Bender Ball, yoga mat

BEGIN: Begin on the hands and knees, placing the right hand on the ball. Next, lightly press into the ball. Initiate the exercise with a long straight spine and keep the abdominals engaged to protect the back. Place the hands the width of the shoulder. Next, lift the left knee off of the floor for a more advanced movement. Repeat 10 times on each side.

PURPOSE: To strengthen the muscles surrounding the shoulder and giving an option of not performing a push-up on the floor.

1

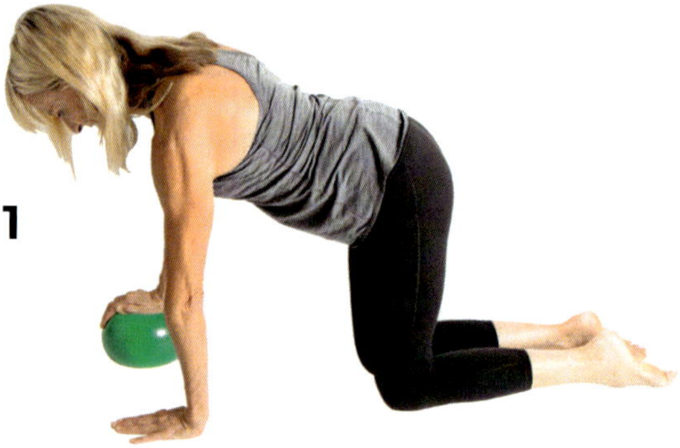

2

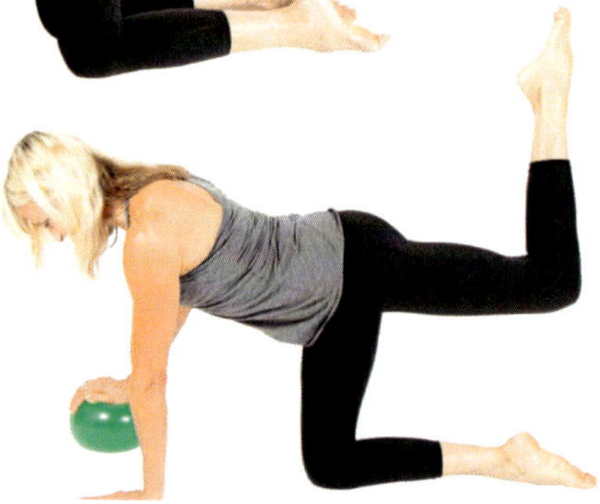

MOVEMENT 29

BRIDGE WITH BENDER BALL

Bridging is an essential exercise to strengthen the glutes and hamstrings. Very important not to squeeze your glutes as it is not necessary but rather than, focus on the core and neutral spine. Think of floating up and when you do lengthen the front of the thighs. Breathe through the exercise as it will help to activate and stabilize the core and spine.

WHAT YOU NEED: Bender Ball, yoga mat

BEGIN: (1) Begin lying on your back with the ball in between the knees lift the hips in a neutral position and spine until you feel your hamstrings, inner thighs and glutes engage, lower back down repeat 10 times. **(2)** Begin in the same position, lift the hips and take the right foot off of the floor for more intensity and balance. Keep the hips parallel. Lower and repeat on the left 10 times. **(3)** Begin with the feet on the ball (most advanced). Lift the hips until the hamstrings engage and lower 10 times.

PURPOSE: To strengthen the hamstrings, glutes and inner thighs.

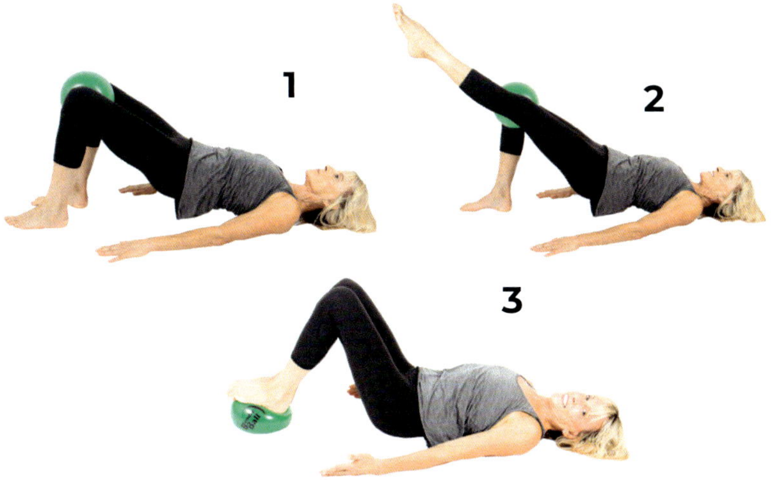

MOVEMENT 30

BALANCE AND HAMSTRING STRETCH WITH BENDER BALL

This is not only a great core exercise but it will challenge your balance as well if you choose to take the hands off the floor. Also if your hamstrings are tight (as they are for most people) begin by placing the ball under the tailbone; this is a wonderful way to stretch the hamstrings.

WHAT YOU NEED: Bender Ball, yoga mat

BEGIN: (1) Begin on your back and place the ball under your tailbone. Next lift the feet off of the floor with knees bent, alternating tapping the toes to the floor and focusing on your core and breath Repeat 10 times. **(2)** Extend both knees to lengthen and stretch the hamstrings. Take your hands off of the mat for a balance challenge, or simply keep the knees extended for a stretch. Simply stay there and take deep breaths.

PURPOSE: To lengthen the hamstrings and work on core balance.

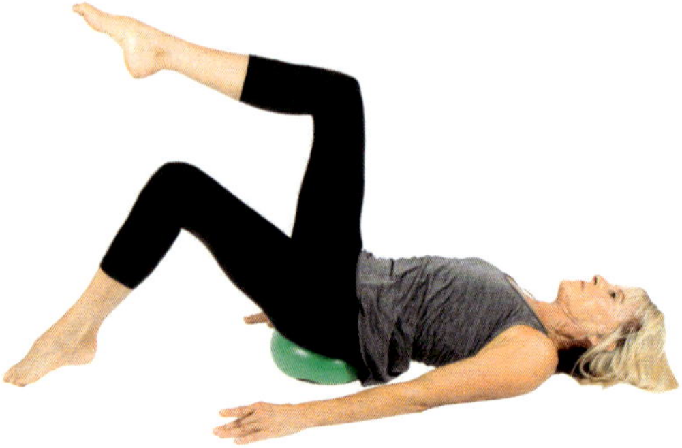

1

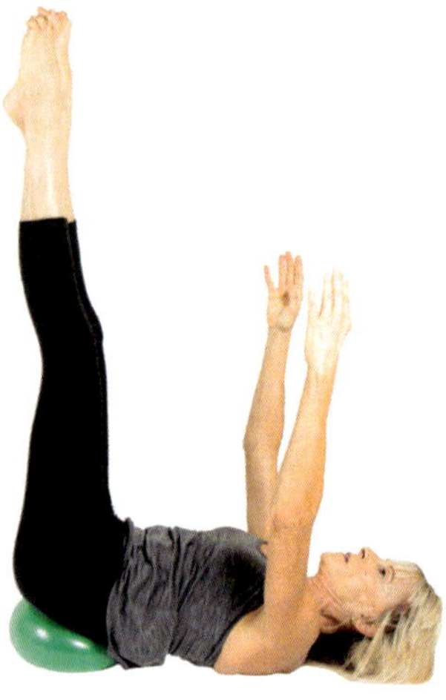

2

MOVEMENT 31

HIP FLEXOR AND STRETCH WITH BENDER BALL

This is a go-to stretch for many different issues such as back or knee pain, as it lengthens the hip flexors while you are relaxing on your back. I suggest doing this movement every day if you want to feel an immediate difference in your body. We carry so much stress in our hips that this is a welcome relief.

WHAT YOU NEED: Bender Ball, yoga mat

BEGIN: Begin on your back, lift your hips and place half of the ball under your right hip. You will want the left one on the mat. Your right hip is elevated slightly. Reach the right arm over the head and think of lengthening the body while you straighten the right and then the left knee, while keeping your heels on the ground. Stay in this stretch one to two minutes, taking deep breaths. Repeat on the left.

PURPOSE: To lengthen the hip flexors in a supine position to relieve back and or knee pain.

1

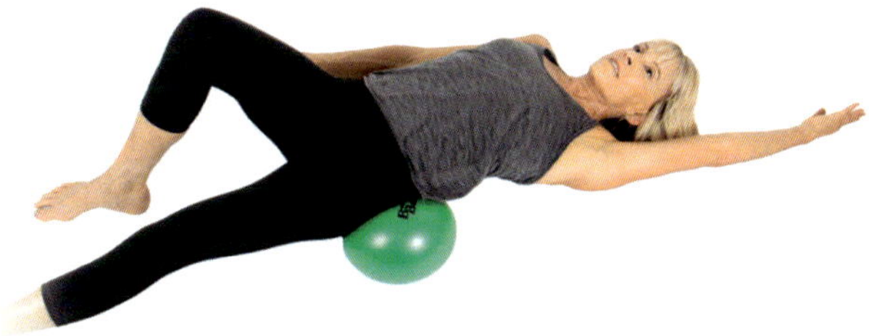

2

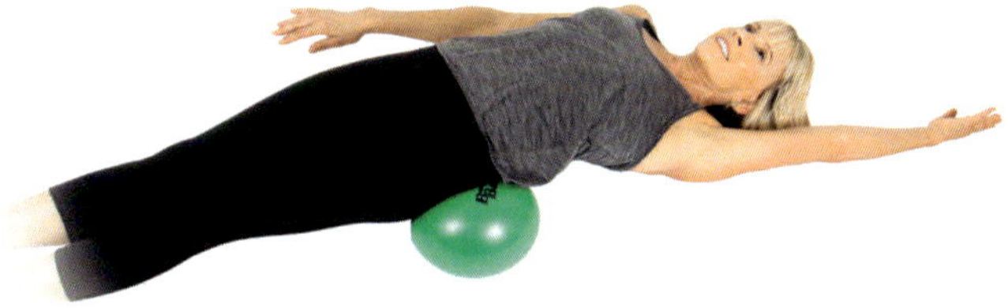

MOVEMENT 32

ARM/SHOULDER STRENGTHENING WITH TUBING

This exercise will define and strengthen your shoulders and triceps for ageless looking arms. Just utilizing tubing is a quick and efficient way to train your body more efficiently and in less time. Keep the resistance the entire time and you will most definitely feel and see the difference!

WHAT YOU NEED: Tubing with handles

BEGIN: Begin by wrapping the tube around your waist and hold the handles. Bend your knees into a small squat. Extend the shoulders behind you and engage your triceps. Keep pressing into the tubing with small ranges of motion for at least 10 times and repeat if you choose.

PURPOSE: To strengthen and lengthen the back of the shoulder and triceps.

1

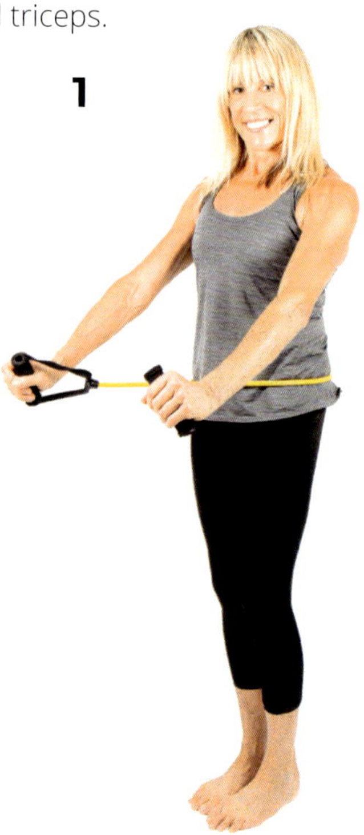

2

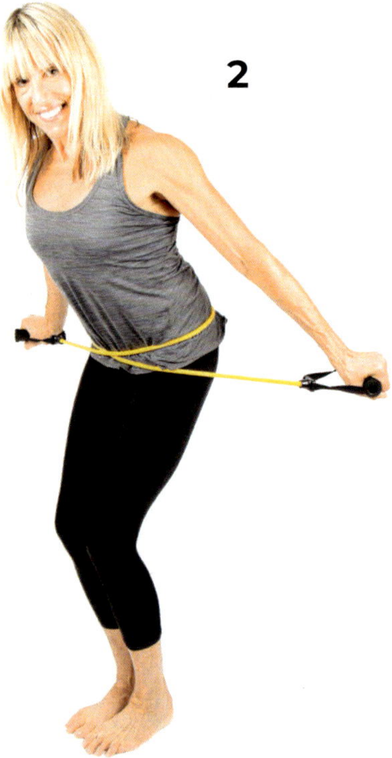

MOVEMENT 33

UPPER BODY ROW AND SIDE LUNGE WITH TUBING

This exercise will define your shoulders, strengthen the legs and give you an ageless body, using tubing for efficiency. It will strengthen the core as well.

WHAT YOU NEED: Tubing with handles

BEGIN: (1) Begin by wrapping the tube around the right foot for security. Have your feet wider than hip width. **(2)** Flex the left knee into a side lunge while keeping the right one straight. Flex the elbows to initiate a bicep curl while you are lunging to the side, and repeat 10 times. **(3)** Flex the left knee into a side lunge again. Pull the tube upward toward the chest, to work your shoulder. Repeat 10 times and repeat on the left.

PURPOSE: To strengthen and lengthen the muscles of the arm and thighs.

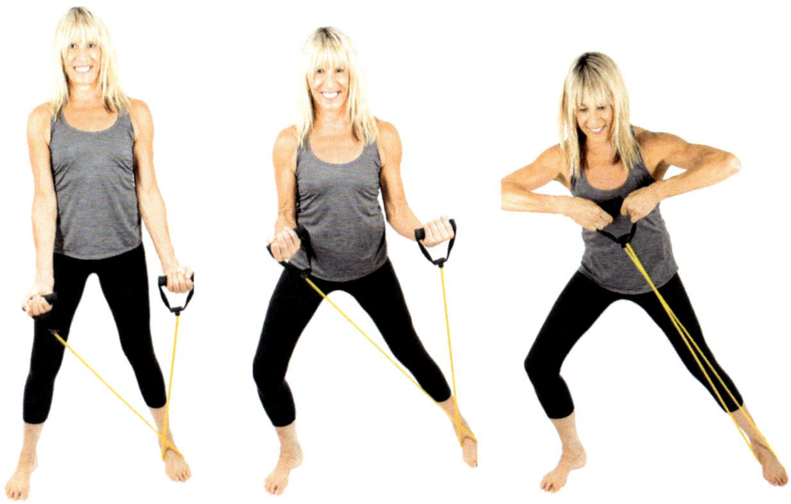

1 2 3

MOVEMENT 34

UPPER BODY ROW WITH TUBING

This exercise will define and sculpt the front of the shoulders by using tubing, which keeps the tension on the shoulders for best results.

WHAT YOU NEED: Tubing with handles

BEGIN: Begin by wrapping the tubing under the right foot for security and lunge back. Next, reach the arms to shoulder height in front of you, and return. Repeat on the left 10 times.

PURPOSE: To train the chest and glutes.

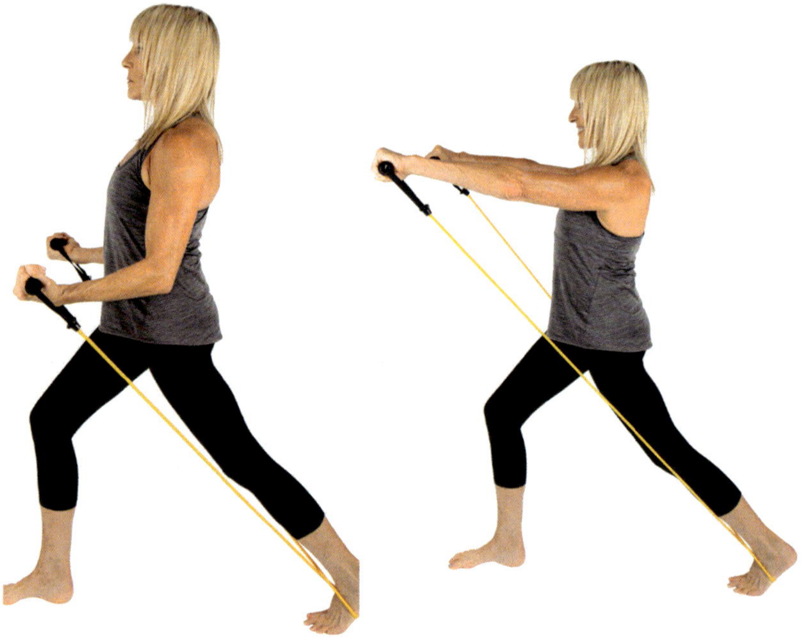

1 2

MOVEMENT 35

STANDING BALANCE HIP LIFT AND ROW WITH TUBING

This exercise will increase balance, strengthen the arms and shoulders, lengthen the hamstrings for an ageless functional body Balance is crucial but so is flexibility and strength, so you have all in this movement. If you feel your balance is compromised, just lift and lower the foot back to the floor in a small range of motion. Don't forget to stand tall and activate your supporting side.

WHAT YOU NEED: Tubing with handles

BEGIN: (1) Begin by wrapping the tube around the right foot. Next lift the left foot off of the floor. Think of lifting and engaging through the right side of the body while activating your hip for balance. Pull the tube upward toward the chest to work the shoulders 10 times. Repeat on the other side. **(2)** Next keep the tube around the right foot and lift it off of the floor. You will now be balancing on the left side. Only lift the right leg to maintain your balance and feel the hamstring engage. Hold the handles in front of you as it will create a bit of resistance, and repeat 10 times. Repeat on the other side. **(3)** Same position as above but with an option to do a bicep curl.

PURPOSE: To strengthen the deltoids and the biceps, to work on balance on the supporting side, and lengthen the hamstrings.

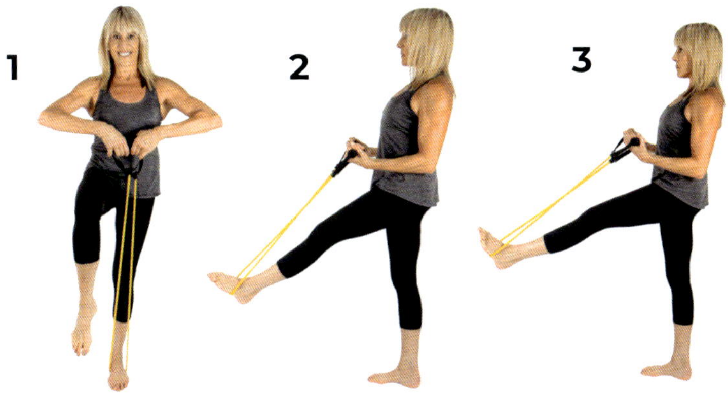

MOVEMENT 36

STANDING BALANCE

This movement works multiple areas from the outer thigh to the shoulder while balancing, all of which are important to strengthening the ageless body for multiple tasks. By using tubing you can train efficiently. Remember, the more you think of lifting and balancing on the supporting side, the better the exercise can be performed.

WHAT YOU NEED: Tubing with handles

BEGIN: Begin by wrapping the tube around the right foot. Hold the right handle on your waist and the left handle out to the side of the body. Next, lift the right hip to the side, focusing on your outer thighs and balance. Repeat 10 times on each side.

PURPOSE: To increase balance and strengthen the side of the hip and shoulder.

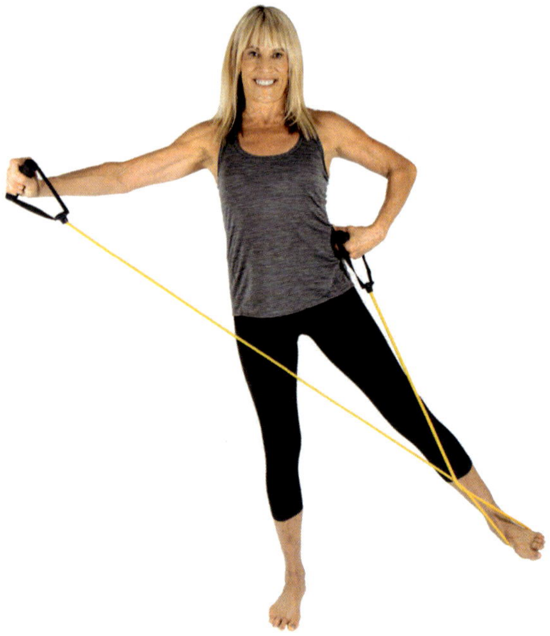

MOVEMENT 37

SEATED CORE WITH BENDER BALL AND GLIDING DISC (HANDHELD WEIGHTS OR TUBING)

This core exercise will strengthen your core efficiently without ever compromising the back or neck. By adding in discs, tubing or weights to the ball, your equipment is similar to Pilates equipment. You will find the intensity and efficiency of this exercise takes less time and better than crunches will ever be! Make sure that when you do lean back over the ball you never feel pain. Only the front of the body will quiver, and you may fatigue quickly.

WHAT YOU NEED: Bender Ball, Gliding discs, tubing with handles, hand weights

BEGIN: Begin seated on the mat. Wedge the Bender Ball directly behind the low back and hips (bunny tail). Next, place your heels on the discs. Slowly raise both arms over the shoulders, extend the upper back while you straighten your knees. Focus on moving slowly, then return. Make sure to breathe and engage your core. You can hold weights or tubing for more intensity. Repeat 10 times.

PURPOSE: To lengthen and strengthen the front of the body's core while protecting the back.

1

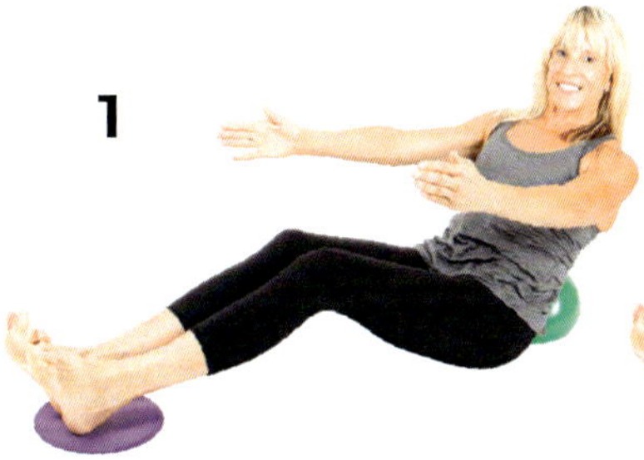

2

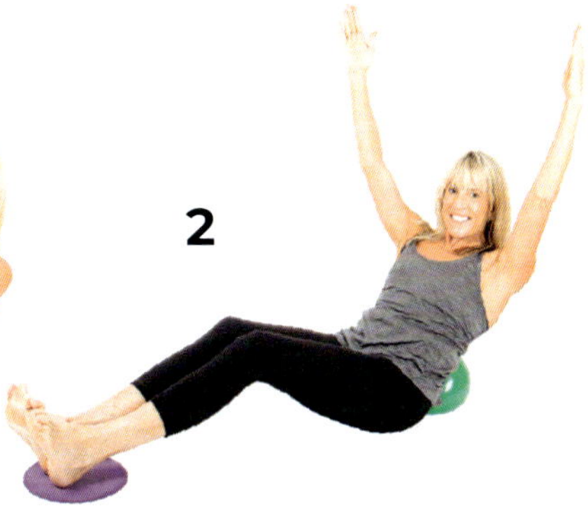

MOVEMENT 38

SIDE-LYING CORE

This is the ultimate waist-definer while protecting your back. By adding the discs it allows you to move freely on the ball and feel your core (primarily the obliques) engage. If you are an active individual, this will improve your game and your ageless body!

WHAT YOU NEED: Bender Ball, Gliding disc

BEGIN: Begin side lying. Place the ball between your right hip and ribs. Next, place your right hand on the disc. Slowly start to slide the disc away from you. Next, reach your left arm over your right shoulder as though you were reaching for something while side bending. Feel your core engage. Return to the beginning position. Repeat 10 times on each side.

PURPOSE: To strengthen and define the obliques and core.

1

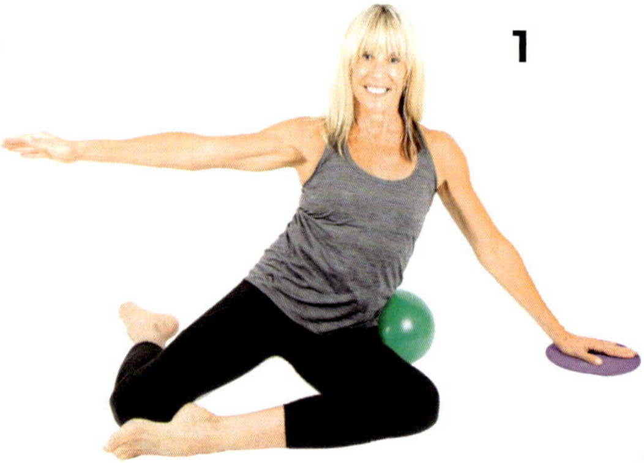

2

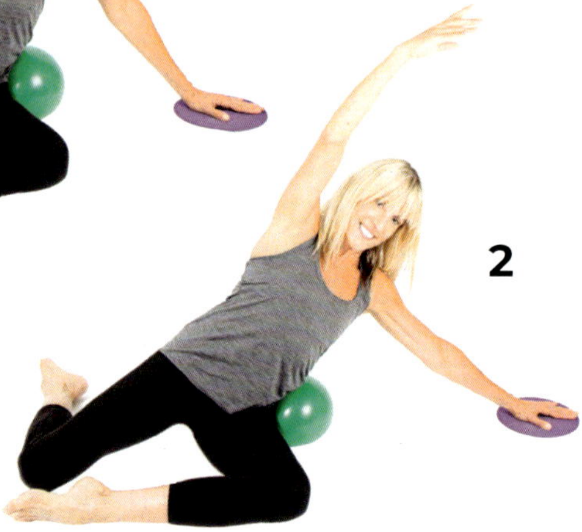

MOVEMENT 39

RESTORE THE BOTTOM OF THE FEET WITH ROLLER

This is a great way to start or end the day with a foot massage. Our feet are so sensitive and this will help to restore balance, increase stimulation, and help the feet perform better, which is a direct link to the rest of the body. Using the foam roller is different than the tennis ball and is a great compliment to that massage.

WHAT YOU NEED: Roller, yoga mat

BEGIN: Begin standing or sitting placing the roller under the right foot. Press the arch of the foot on the roller and slowly roll from the heels to the toes for about 30 seconds. Move the foot to flex and extend the toes. Compress the arch on the roller and hold for about 30 seconds and take deep breaths. Repeat on the left foot.

PURPOSE: Rolling the fascia helps diminish aches, pain and stiffness, and will increase your flexibility, hydration, blood flow, and range of motion.

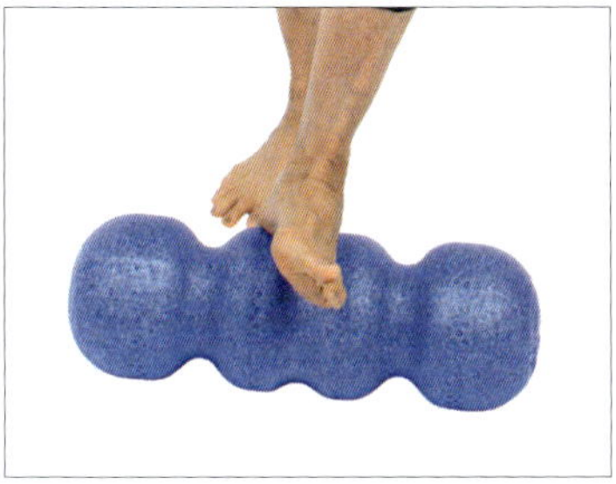

MOVEMENT 40

RESTORE THE CALVES

This is a such a vital massage for tired overworked calves that result from uncomfortable shoes, standing for long periods, or running, just to name a few. The calves are sensitive and there will be areas using a roller that may feel more intense than the tennis ball. Make sure to breathe through the intense part of the rolling as it will help decrease any discomfort.

WHAT YOU NEED: Roller, yoga mat

BEGIN: Begin seated upright with your hands (or hand) behind you for support on the mat, and place the right calf on the roller. Slowly bend and flex the right knee rolling inward and outward or side to side. You can place your left leg on top of the right, which will add more pressure, for approximately one minute. Repeat on the left.

PURPOSE: To massage the calves for better flexibility and mobility.

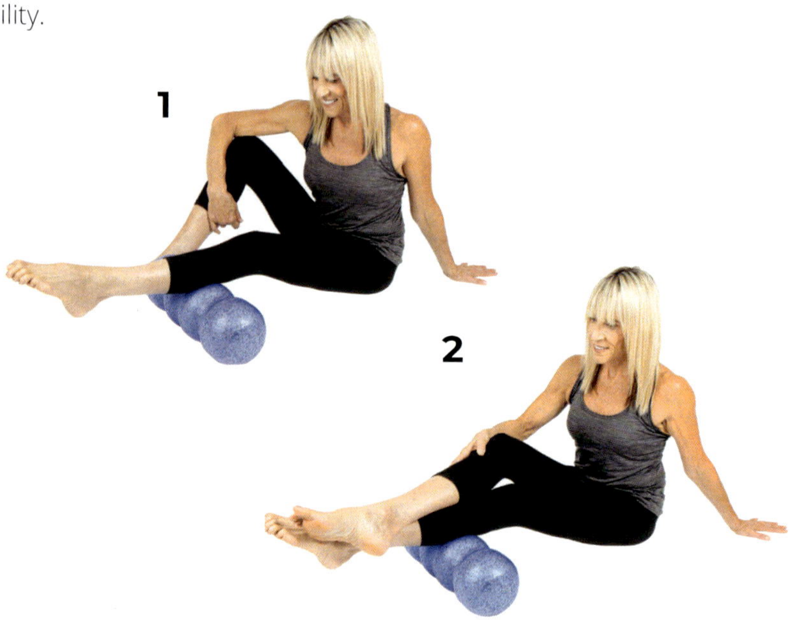

MOVEMENT 41

RESTORE THE FOREARMS

This is a vital massage for the forearms for anyone who sits at a computer for a long time. Take a break and give those forearms some love! We also use the arms more than we think by lifting, pushing, pulling, etc. You can do this as a break from your computer work or even sitting watching TV.

WHAT YOU NEED: Roller, yoga mat

BEGIN: Begin in a seated position either on a mat or a chair placing the roller on your thighs. Next place your forearms on the roller and slowly roll back and forth while turning your palms upward and downward for as long as it feels good to you.

PURPOSE: To help relieve tension in the forearms especially if you are sitting over a computer!

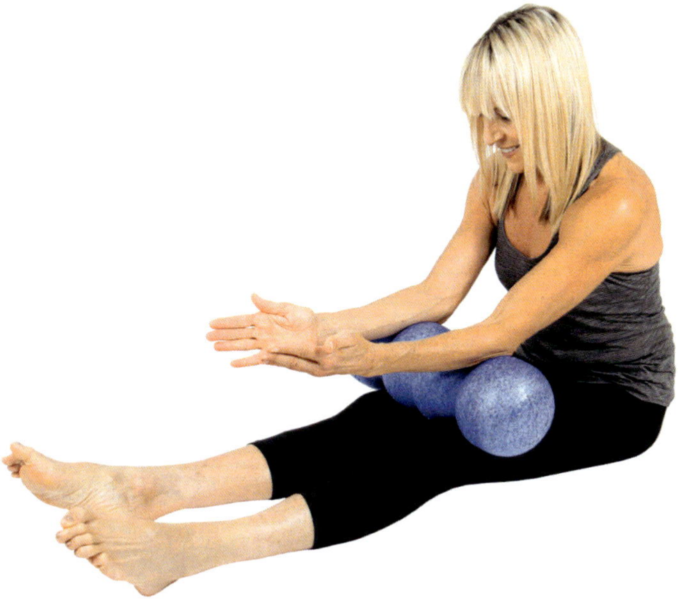

MOVEMENT 42

RESTORE THE SHINS

Your shins can get tired from standing or running (shin splints). This exercise will help you to have happier shins that will be in less pain and function better. If you find that your shins are very fatigued you will also may want to check the quality of your shoes to see if they are placing your feet in a compromised position (especially if you're running). If you are also one of those with thicker skin, this one can be a bit painful so you can always place a towel on the roller for padding.

WHAT YOU NEED: Roller, yoga mat

BEGIN: (1) Begin on your hands or forearms and the right shin on the roller. Extend the left hip with the foot on the mat. Next slowly massage the right shin by moving the knee forward and back for as long as it feels good to you. **(2)** For more intensity place both shins on the roller while either on the hands or forearms You then will want to slowly roll forward and back. Make sure you engage your core. **(3)** You can also do this on the forearms if you experience wrist pain.

PURPOSE: This movement is essential for runners with shin splints and or sore shins.

1

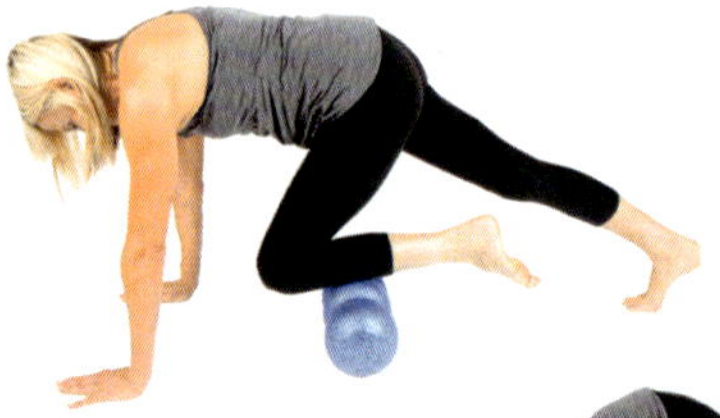

2

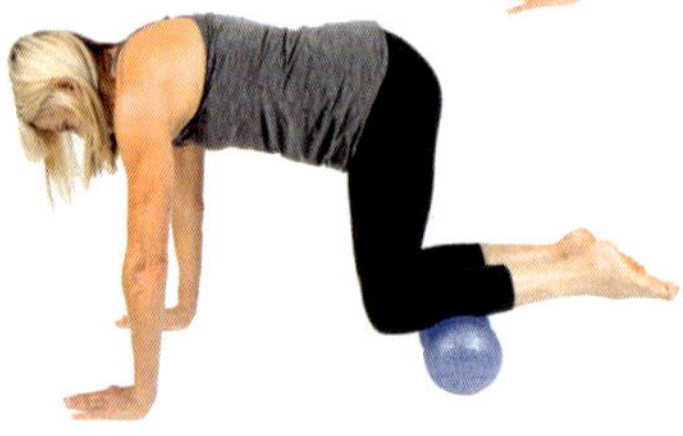

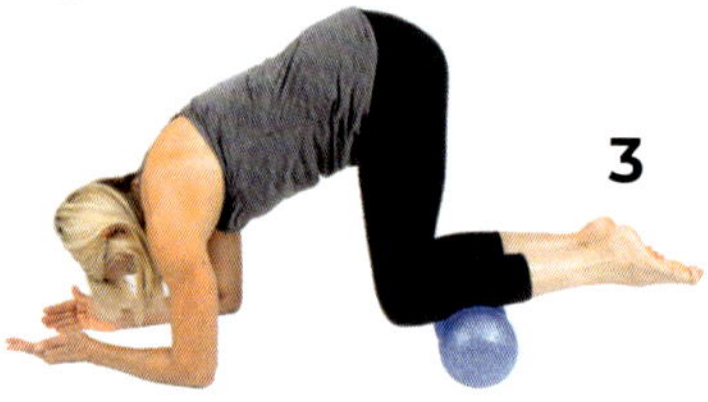

3

MOVEMENT 43

RESTORE THE THIGHS

Your thighs (quads) need massage more than any other part of the body as they are working all the time for so many movements such as climbing stars. This is a must-do massage for healthy ageless legs. Also, when we perform squats the quads will be sore and tight, as with running. Massage not only helps with function but also allows them to become stronger and more efficient.

WHAT YOU NEED: Roller, yoga mat

BEGIN: Begin on your forearms and the thighs on the roller. Slowly start to move forward and back while bending and extending the knees. You may want to find spots that are sensitive and spend some extra time on them by just holding your position. Each person is different, and you may want to take more time on your thighs. Remember this is where you are never in a rush and take deep breaths on the painful areas so that it becomes more tolerable. The more you do this the easier it will become and even daily is not too much for the hard-working quads.

PURPOSE: To massage and release the tension in the thighs.

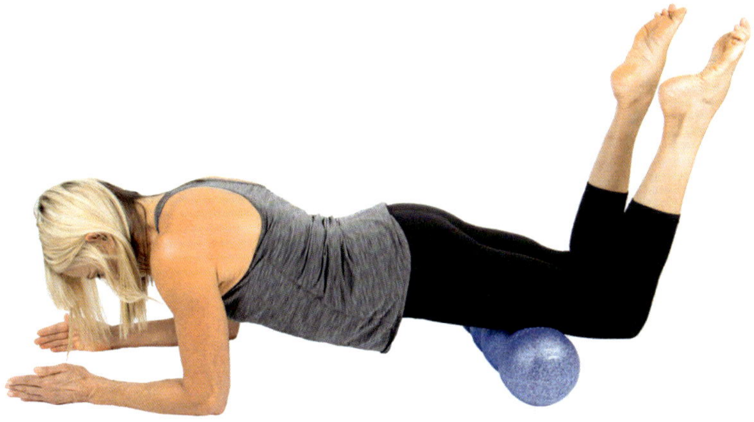

MOVEMENT 44

RESTORE THE INNER THIGH

The inner thigh is not only sensitive, it's also often forgotten in many movement programs. Yet the inner thighs play a big role in the alignment of the hips and knees, so giving them equal attention is a great plan. If you are a runner or cyclist this is an important restorative movement. You will find your performance increased and range of motion as well.

WHAT YOU NEED: Roller, yoga mat

BEGIN: Begin on your forearms and place the roller under the inner thigh between the knee and the hip, not too close to the groin. Slowly move the roller forward and back to massage the inner thigh area. Again, it's a very sensitive area. You can extend the knee for a different experience. Remember to breathe.

PURPOSE: To restore the inner part of the thigh.

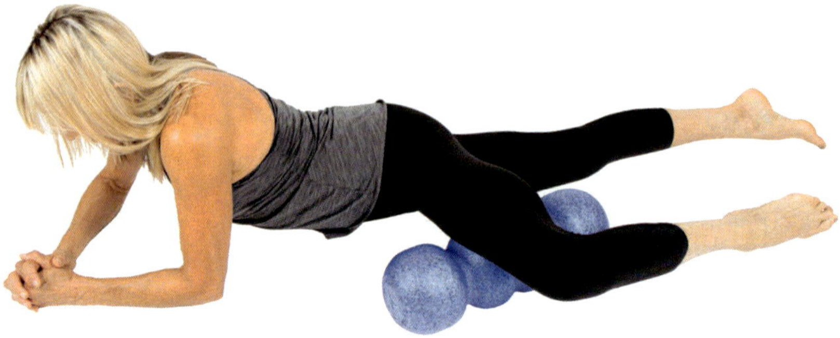

MOVEMENT 45

RESTORE THE GLUTES

As we all know, the glutes love a good massage. We sit, squat, run, walk, and demand a lot from our poor butt! This is a daily must do to keep your glutes happy, functional, and pain-free. Every time we get up and down the glutes work, and sitting is the worst thing we can do to our body for long periods—we were not designed to sit. Make sure to breathe and if you choose to lean a bit to the side when doing this movement, you may find it to be painful as it is near the sciatic nerve.

WHAT YOU NEED: Roller, yoga mat

BEGIN: Begin by sitting on the roller upright. Place the hands to the side for balance. Next roll forward and back slowly. You can lean to one side for more intensity or stay on a sensitive area. You may want to take time and relax while sitting on the roller.

PURPOSE: This is an essential movement and massage; we all sit, and the glutes get sore.

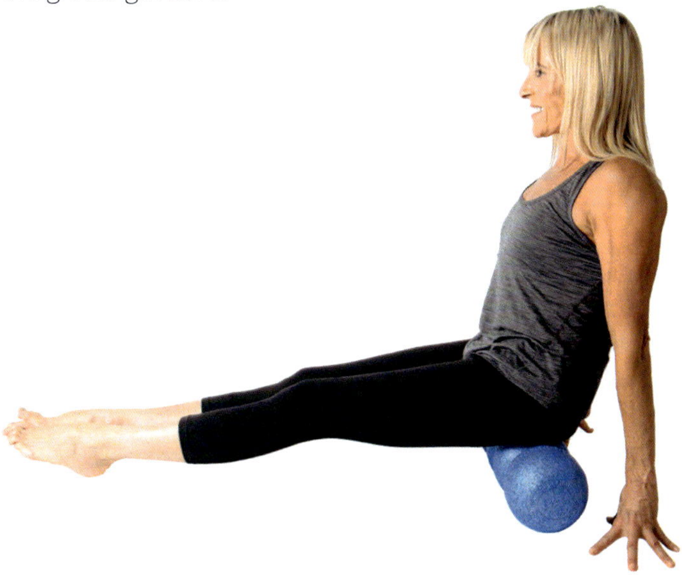

MOVEMENT 46

RESTORE THE HAMSTRINGS

The hamstrings, like the glutes, can get very tight and dysfunctional from sitting, so this is also a must-do movement after a long day—or even before you train your legs. Also, hamstrings are one of those muscle groups that are one of the first to experience an injury from sports like skiing. But when cared for, massaged, and lengthened, they will stay ageless. And as always, breathe through the movement.

WHAT YOU NEED: Roller, yoga mat

BEGIN: Begin sitting on the roller, upright with your hands behind you. Next cross the left leg over the right while on the roller. Slowly roll forward and back. You can also lean from side to side to feel other areas of the hamstrings. You may want to take your time here to restore the hamstrings. Repeat on the other leg. Stay on the painful areas as long as needed as they are sensitive.

PURPOSE: To stretch the hamstring muscles.

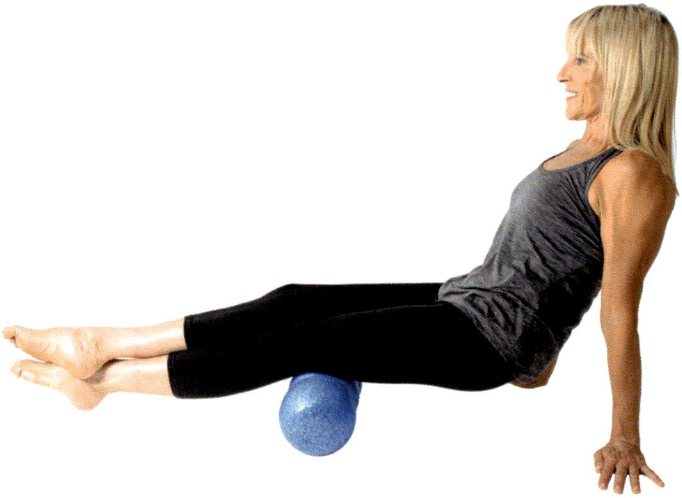

MOVEMENT 47

RESTORE THE OUTER THIGHS

The outer thighs (we know it as the IT band) get tight. It is best to roll above the IT band and not directly on it, as it is very sensitive. It's also been known to keep the hip and knee aligned. Runners and cyclists typically have outer thighs that need restoring through massage. This will keep your hips and knees happy for an ageless body and everlasting performance. Breathe deeply when rolling and massaging the outer thigh.

WHAT YOU NEED: Roller, yoga mat

BEGIN: Begin by sitting on the roller with the right hip. Cross the left in front for balance with your foot on the floor. Next roll and move onto the front of the hip and massage slowly on the roller, staying off the IT band (you will know if you are on it due to how painful it can be). Repeat on the left. Take as much time and sit on the areas that are sensitive for at least ten seconds, and breathe.

PURPOSE: To restore the outer part of the thigh as it can get very tight from training, sitting, and many daily activities.

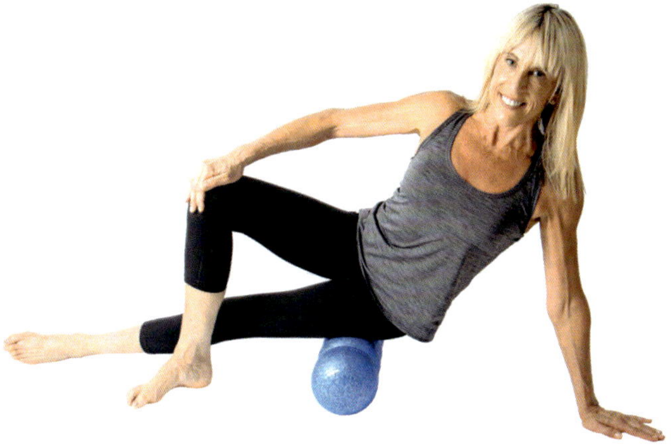

MOVEMENT 48

RESTORE THE UPPER BACK AND SHOULDERS

This is a must massage for anyone under stress, or from sitting for long hours at a desk. Your upper back and shoulders carry so much on them on emotionally and physically that this is a way to de-stress and feel ageless again! It will also improve posture and overall well-being Stay as long as needed and take deep breaths here for maximum relaxation.

WHAT YOU NEED: Roller, yoga mat

BEGIN: (1) Begin with the roller under the mid back and the shoulders with your hips on the mat. Hold and support your head and neck. **(2)** Slowly flex from side to side so the roller can get in between the shoulder blades. Do as many as you need for each side of the body (for more intensity you can lift the hips). You may find that one side is more tender than the other.

PURPOSE: To take away tension we all have in the upper back.

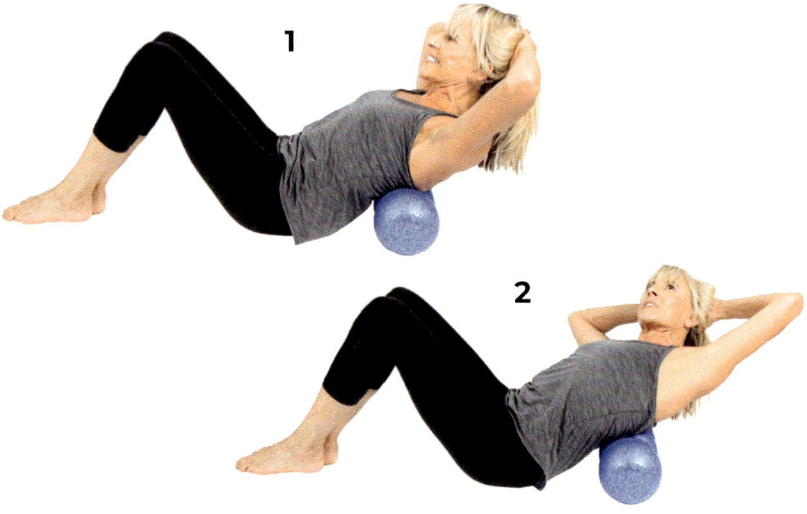

MOVEMENT 49

RESTORE THE NECK

We all know the saying, "I have a pain in my neck!" This is a massage that will relieve the tension in your neck and help you to sleep better. And we know when we do not have tension in the neck we look and feel younger! We carry a lot of stress in the neck and it can be debilitating. Grab some lavender oil and take at least three to five minutes here to allow your stress melt away.

WHAT YOU NEED: Roller, yoga mat

BEGIN: Begin lying on your mat and place the roller under the neck like a pillow. Next close your eyes and slowly turn your head from right to left and relax. Allow your body to feel heavy and take deep breaths with this relaxing movement.

PURPOSE: To release stress, which is necessary to stay ageless.

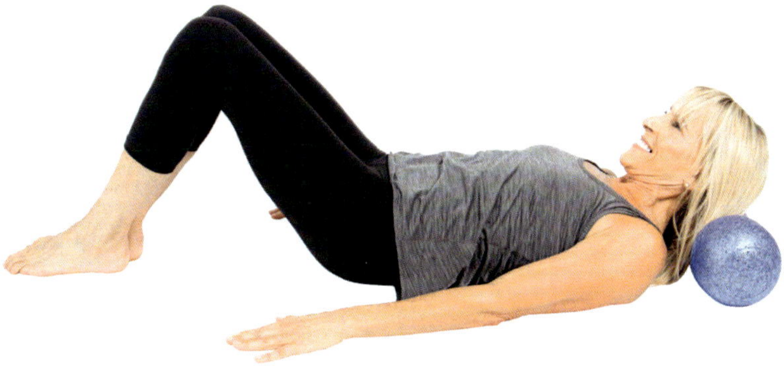

MOVEMENT 50

RESTORE THE FEET

Take a load off your feet and back with this soothing massage for the feet. This helps relax tired feet. It's best to do before going to bed (do the standing massage with the tennis ball in the morning to get you going).

WHAT YOU NEED: Roller, yoga mat

BEGIN: Begin lying on your back on the mat. Place your feet on the roller and roll them back and forth, massaging the bottoms and sides. Take as long as needed to feel your feet relax and unwind.

PURPOSE: To massage the bottom of the feet for better elasticity, mobility and balance.

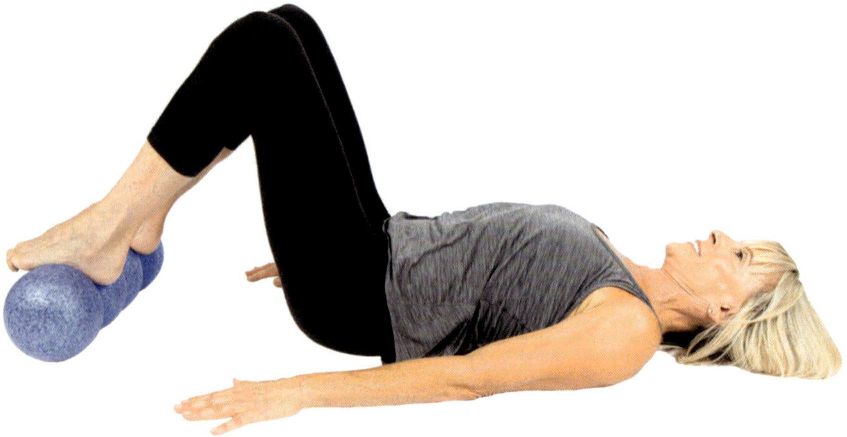

I Am Ageless Now Combinations

1. Movement 1: FOOT MASSAGE
2. Movement 2: CALF MASSAGE
3. Movement 3: OUTER THIGH MASSAGE
4. Movement 4: GLUTE MASSAGE
5. Movement 11: STRETCH YOUR CALVES
6. Movement 12: STRETCH THE FRONT OF YOUR HIPS

Restore Your Back

1. Movement 1: FOOT MASSAGE
2. Movement 9: MASSAGE YOUR NECK
3. Movement 13: STRETCH THE BACK OF YOUR HIPS AND LEGS
4. Movement 14: STRETCH THE SIDE OF YOUR HIPS
5. Movement 48: RESTORE THE UPPER BACK AND SHOULDERS
6. Movement 49: RESTORE THE NECK

Restore Your Hips

1. Movement 1: FOOT MASSAGE
2. Movement 3: OUTER THIGH MASSAGE
3. Movement 4: GLUTE MASSAGE
4. Movement 12: STRETCH THE FRONT OF YOUR HIPS
5. Movement 13: STRETCH THE BACK OF YOUR HIPS AND LEGS
6. Movement 14: STRETCH THE SIDE OF YOUR HIPS

Morning Glory

1. Movement 1: FOOT MASSAGE
2. Movement 11: STRETCH YOUR CALVES
3. Movement 12: STRETCH THE FRONT OF YOUR HIPS

4. Movement 13: STRETCH THE BACK OF YOUR HIPS AND LEGS
5. Movement 16: LUNGING WITH GLIDING DISC OR PAPER PLATE
6. Movement 25: SEATED CORE WITH BENDER BALL

Morning Energy Boost

1. Movement 1: FOOT MASSAGE
2. Movement 11: STRETCH YOUR CALVES
3. Movement 20: BENDER BALL SQUATS/STAGGERED/BALANCE
4. Movement 23: BENDER BALL LUNGES
5. Movement 24: BENDER BALL LUNGES TO THE SIDE
6. Movement 25: SEATED CORE WITH BENDER BALL

Afternoon Stretch

1. Movement 20: BENDER BALL SQUATS/STAGGERED/BALANCE
2. Movement 24: BENDER BALL LUNGES TO THE SIDE
3. Movement 25: SEATED CORE WITH BENDER BALL
4. Movement 33: UPPER BODY EXERCISE ROW/SIDE LUNGE WITH TUBING
5. Movement 34: UPPER BODY ROW WITH TUBING
6. Movement 36: STANDING BALANCE

Core and More

1. Movement 37: SEATED CORE WITH BENDER BALL AND GLIDING
2. Movement 38: SIDE-LYING CORE
3. Movement 27: HANDS AND KNEES BALANCE WITH BENDER BALL
4. Movement 28: HAND BALANCE WITH BENDER BALL
5. Movement 18: PLANK WITH GLIDING DISC OR PAPER PLATES
6. Movement 17: SKATER WITH GLIDING DISC OR PAPER PLATE

Evening Wind Down

1. Movement 4: GLUTE MASSAGE
2. Movement 13: STRETCH THE BACK OF YOUR HIPS AND LEGS
3. Movement 25: SEATED CORE WITH BENDER BALL
4. Movement 31: HIP FLEXOR & SHOULDER STRETCH WITH BENDER BALL
5. Movement 43: RESTORE THE THIGHS
6. Movement 48: RESTORE THE UPPER BACK AND SHOULDERS

Evening Rest and Relax

1. Movement 39: RESTORE THE BOTTOM OF THE FEET
2. Movement 40: RESTORE THE CALVES
3. Movement 41: RESTORE THE FOREARMS
4. Movement 42: RESTORE THE SHIN
5. Movement 46: RESTORE THE HAMSTRINGS
6. Movement 48: RESTORE THE UPPER BACK AND SHOULDERS

We are not victims of aging, sickness, and death. These are part of scenery, not the seer, who is immune to any form of change. This seer is the spirit, the expression of eternal being.

Deepak Chopra

30-DAY I AM AGELESS NOW TRANSFORMATION

Boost your mindfulness. Increase your good nutrition. Pump up your movement. Become more flexible and fluid.

30-Day Ageless Now Transformation

This 30-day Ageless Now Transformation is set up to help you craft new habits over the next month. And no, you don't have to wait until the first of the month to start. Start now!

It's designed to jump-start your commitment of a new Ageless Now you. It takes discipline and tenacity to transition old habits into new ones. The transformation pages include selected exercises for each day from the movement section, space to record your (possibly new) healthy food choices (or a daily record of your nutrition), and space to write a mantra or affirmation to do each day. There's also a chart to keep track of your hydration. If you can, set aside the same time each day, with the fewest possible distractions to do this work. It's hard—we all have distractions. If you are a morning person, you'll probably find this is a great way to start your day.

If you can, find a specific place that can become yours and yours alone to do the 30-Day Transformation. Some days you may want to do your movements outside, where you can breathe in fresh air and even add in a cardio walk or bike ride. These 30 days are designed to give you a new perspective of your life and an indication of how a few small changes can help you live with less pain, more energy, and feel fit for life.

Be yourself today. You look beautiful like that.

Change is a challenge but necessary for growth at any age! Here are a few questions to ask yourself, to help you see if you are ready to begin the Ageless Now Transformation:

- Will you dedicate 10 to 20 minutes every day to making a positive behavioral outcome?
- Will you dedicate 10 to 20 minutes every day to making a positive physical outcome?
- Will you dedicate at least 5 minutes a day to quiet and reflective time, such as meditation?
- Will you commit to trying different (maybe some new) nutritional choices every day?
- Will you decrease watching TV?
- Will you decrease alcohol consumption?
- Will you decrease caffeine consumption?
- Will you decrease poor food choices such as fried foods, sugar, processed carbs, etc.?
- Will you decrease drinking sodas, energy drinks, etc.?
- Will you take time to write down your goals, affirmations and what you want out of your life?

If you answered yes to all of these questions you are ready to rock! If you answered yes to 7 out of 10, then you may need to re-think what you have to work on. And if you said yes to fewer than 5, what do you need to work on to make this commitment? What is stopping you from the life you deserve? Don't self-sabotage your life. Our time here on this earth is short, so don't make it just an audition—make it the performance!

We encourage you not to get frustrated if you don't progress as quickly as you'd like. Your path may not be a straight line (in fact, it probably won't). You'll be able to look back over your entries and see where you zigged where you could have zagged.

Please note we said *could have*, not *should have*. There are no "shoulds" here. This is your work and you need to do it in the way that feels right for you. As long as you keep your goal in sight—remember why you're doing this, why you want more movement, better health, and a happier life—you will become who you intend to be. Successful people don't give up after one bad day. It's just a day, and tomorrow is a fresh opportunity.

This work is not difficult, but you do have to DO the work. Every day.

As you go through this 30-day Transformation, use the mantras for every movement. We've suggested one mantra on each day, and there's space for you to add your own. Repeat the mantras out loud. If you are self-conscious, say them out loud anyway. This is part of how you retrain your brain to speak to yourself with love and respect.

If there are people in your space who make you uncomfortable or self-conscious as you begin your new journey, invite them to leave while you focus on yourself. You're worth it. Visualize yourself as the person you want to become. You are not too old, and it's not too late. See yourself as a person who takes action each day and creates the life she/he wants. We can't understate the importance of having a positive mindset with your new activities, along with mindful breathing.

One good way to stay in touch with how you're feeling is to do a mindful body scan. Do it in the morning to boost your day and at the end of the day to reflect. If there's a point during the day when you're anxious or upset, repeat the body scan.

Begin by sitting or lying down. Take a few deep breaths. Consciously feel how your breath enters and leaves your lungs. Continue mindful breathing and focus your attention on one part of your body, beginning with your toes. Continue up the body to the next part of your body, paying attention to how each part feels as you breathe deeply. This exercise helps put you in a mindful state and helps you notice how your body feels in different situations.

HOW TO USE THE TRANSFORMATION PAGES

On the following pages you will find space to record your mantras, activities, mindful activities, nutrition and hydration, and fitness goals.

Each day you'll also find:

- Suggested **exercise combinations** using the movements from section 4. The combinations are designed to help you cross train to make sure you keep all parts of your body fit and flexible.
- Space to note your nutrition—what you've eaten during the day. Make sure to add **higher-level nutrition** to your diet to help keep your body Ageless Now.
- A **mantra** to get you started, along with space to write your own.
- A spot to keep track of your **hydration**.

Everything begins and ends in your own mind. Whatever you give power to has power over you - if you allow it.

Mantra

I am fearless.

Your own mantra(s):

I AM AGELESS NOW

date day 1 **30-DAY TRANSFORMATION**

Today's suggested purposeful and intentional movements: Foot massage (1) Calf massage (2) Stretch your calves (11) Stretch the front of your hips (12)

What else did you do? How did it make you feel?

Today's higher-level nutrition:

Mindful breathing and body scan:

HYDRATION

If your path demands you walk through hell, walk as if you own the place.

Mantra

I am worthy of the blessings coming my way.

Your own mantra(s):

date day 2 **30-DAY TRANSFORMATION**

Today's suggested purposeful and intentional movement: Foot massage (1) Stretch the back of the hips (13) Stretch the side of the hips (14) Bender Ball squat (22)

What else did you do? How did it make you feel?

Today's higher-level nutrition:

Mindful breathing and body scan:

HYDRATION

Invest in your mind. Invest in your health. Invest in yourself.

Mantra

I am a miracle.

Your own mantra(s):

date day 3 **30-DAY TRANSFORMATION**

Today's suggested purposeful and intentional movement: Skater with gliding (17) Plank with gliding (18) Lengthen the and stretch your hips in all directions (15) Seated core (25)

What else did you do? How did it make you feel?

Today's higher-level nutrition:

Mindful breathing and body scan:

HYDRATION

Follow your soul. It knows the way.

Mantra

I am well-balanced and centered.

Your own mantra(s):

I AM AGELESS NOW

date   day 4   **30-DAY TRANSFORMATION**

Today's suggested purposeful and intentional movement: Restore your feet (39) Restore your calves (40) Restore your shins (42) Restore your thighs (43)

What else did you do? How did it make you feel?

Today's higher-level nutrition:

Mindful breathing and body scan:

HYDRATION

You have the power within you to rise above anything that seeks to bring you down.

Mantra

I am amazing.

Your own mantra(s):

I AM AGELESS NOW

date day 5 **30-DAY TRANSFORMATION**

Today's suggested purposeful and intentional movement: Arm/shoulder strengthening with tubing (32) Upper body row and side lunge with tubing (33) Side lying core (38) Seated core (37)

What else did you do? How did it make you feel?

Today's higher-level nutrition:

Mindful breathing and body scan:

HYDRATION

The biggest mistake you can ever make is being too afraid to make one.

Mantra

I am more than enough.

Your own mantra(s):

date day 6 **30-DAY TRANSFORMATION**

Today's suggested purposeful and intentional movement: Balance and hamstring stretch (30) Hip flexor stretch (31) Restore the upper back and shoulders (48) Restore neck (49)

What else did you do? How did it make you feel?

Today's higher-level nutrition:

Mindful breathing and body scan:

HYDRATION

It's never too late for a new beginning, a new you, a new life.

Mantra

I am trusting the journey.

Your own mantra(s):

I AM AGELESS NOW

date day 7 **30-DAY TRANSFORMATION**

Today's suggested purposeful and intentional movement: Bender Ball lunges (24) Bender Ball lunges in all directions (25) Hand balance (28) Bridge (29)

What else did you do? How did it make you feel?

Today's higher-level nutrition:

Mindful breathing and body scan:

HYDRATION

You talk to yourself more than you talk to anyone else. Make sure you say the right things.

Mantra

I am proud of who I am becoming.

Your own mantra(s):

I AM AGELESS NOW

date

day 8 **30-DAY TRANSFORMATION**

Today's suggested purposeful and intentional movement: Restore the glutes (44) Restore the outer thigh (46) Restore the inner thigh (47) Restore the shin (42)

What else did you do? How did it make you feel?

Today's higher-level nutrition:

Mindful breathing and body scan:

HYDRATION

You will never have this day again. Make it count.

Mantra

I am fortunate.

Your own mantra(s):

I AM AGELESS NOW

date day 9 **30-DAY TRANSFORMATION**

Today's suggested purposeful and intentional movement: Stretch your calves (11) Stretch your hips in all directions (15) Lunging with gliding (16) Plank with Gliding (19)

What else did you do? How did it make you feel?

Today's higher-level nutrition:

Mindful breathing and body scan:

HYDRATION

It's OK if the only thing you did today was breathe. Try again tomorrow.

Mantra

I am abundant.

Your own mantra(s):

I AM AGELESS NOW

date

day 10 **30-DAY TRANSFORMATION**

Today's suggested purposeful and intentional movement: Hand balance with Bender Ball (28) Side lying with Bender Ball (26) Bridge (29) Hip flexor stretch (31)

What else did you do? How did it make you feel?

Today's higher-level nutrition:

Mindful breathing and body scan:

HYDRATION

Your partner is a reflection of you. Invest wisely.

Mantra

I am full of life.

Your own mantra(s):

I AM AGELESS NOW

date day 11 **30-DAY TRANSFORMATION**

Today's suggested purposeful and intentional movement: Bender Ball lunges to the side (24) Seated core with Bender Ball (25) Lunging with Gliding (16) Plank with Gliding (19)

What else did you do? How did it make you feel?

Today's higher-level nutrition:

Mindful breathing and body scan:

HYDRATION

Surround yourself with people who lift you up.

Mantra

I am comfortable in my own skin.

Your own mantra(s):

I AM AGELESS NOW

date day 12 **30-DAY TRANSFORMATION**

Today's suggested purposeful and intentional movement: Foot massage (1) Calf massage (2) Outer thigh massage (3) Glute massage (4)

What else did you do? How did it make you feel?

Today's higher-level nutrition:

Mindful breathing and body scan:

HYDRATION

Stop shrinking yourself to fit into the places you've long outgrown.

Mantra

I am strong.

Your own mantra(s):

I AM AGELESS NOW

date *day* 13 **30-DAY TRANSFORMATION**

Today's suggested purposeful and intentional movement: Hip flexor massage (5) Massage your neck (9) Bender Ball squats (20) Bender Ball directional lunges (23)

What else did you do? How did it make you feel?

Today's higher-level nutrition:

Mindful breathing and body scan:

HYDRATION

Let's worry less about what could go wrong and start being excited about what could go right.

Mantra

I am willing to ask for help.

Your own mantra(s):

I AM AGELESS NOW

date

day 14 **30-DAY TRANSFORMATION**

Today's suggested purposeful and intentional movement: Bender Ball lunges to the side (24) Hands and knees balance with the Bender Ball (27) Upper body row with tubing (33) Upper body row with tubing (34)

What else did you do? How did it make you feel?

Today's higher-level nutrition:

Mindful breathing and body scan:

HYDRATION

If you don't make time for your wellness, you will be forced to make time for your illness.

Mantra

I am proud of my decisions.

Your own mantra(s):

I AM AGELESS NOW

date day 15 **30-DAY TRANSFORMATION**

Today's suggested purposeful and intentional movement: Side lying core (38) Bender Ball squat with balance (22) Arm/shoulder strengthening with tube (32) Standing balance with tube (35)

What else did you do? How did it make you feel?

Today's higher-level nutrition:

Mindful breathing and body scan:

HYDRATION

Train yourself to see the good in everything. Good things happen. Love is real. We will all be OK.

Mantra

I am joyful.

Your own mantra(s):

I AM AGELESS NOW

date day 16 **30-DAY TRANSFORMATION**

Today's suggested purposeful and intentional movement: Restore the upper back (48) Restore the outer thigh (46) Restore the glutes (44) Restore the neck (49)

What else did you do? How did it make you feel?

Today's higher-level nutrition:

Mindful breathing and body scan:

HYDRATION

Kind words are like honey, sweet to the soul and healing to the bones.

Mantra

I am confident.

Your own mantra(s):

I AM AGELESS NOW

date day 17 **30-DAY TRANSFORMATION**

Today's suggested purposeful and intentional movement: Seated core with Bender Ball (25) Side lying core with Bender Ball (26) Skater with Gliding (17) Plank with Gliding (19)

What else did you do? How did it make you feel?

Today's higher-level nutrition:

Mindful breathing and body scan:

HYDRATION

Be brave. Be silly. Be your own magic. Be present. Be adventurous. Be kind. Be free. Be ageless. Be you.

Mantra

I am kind.

Your own mantra(s):

I AM AGELESS NOW

date

day 18 **30-DAY TRANSFORMATION**

Today's suggested purposeful and intentional movement: Restore your feet (39) Restore your thighs (43) Restore your shin (42) Restore your glutes (44)

What else did you do? How did it make you feel?

Today's higher-level nutrition:

Mindful breathing and body scan:

HYDRATION

Keep calm
and be
Ageless Now.

Mantra

I am grateful.

Your own mantra(s):

I AM AGELESS NOW

date day 19 **30-DAY TRANSFORMATION**

Today's suggested purposeful and intentional movement: Bender Ball squat with Balance (22) Hands and knees balance with Bender Ball (27) Balance and hamstring stretch with Bender Ball (30) Bridge with Bender Ball (29)

What else did you do? How did it make you feel?

Today's higher-level nutrition:

Mindful breathing and body scan:

HYDRATION

Be ageless in the way you think, in what you do, and in how you move.

Mantra

I am beautiful.

Your own mantra(s):

I AM AGELESS NOW

date

day 20 **30-DAY TRANSFORMATION**

Today's suggested purposeful and intentional movement: Hip flexor massage (5) Stretch the front of the hip (12) Glute massage (4) Stretch the back of the hips (13).

What else did you do? How did it make you feel?

Today's higher-level nutrition:

Mindful breathing and body scan:

HYDRATION

Thoughts are things and they have wings.

Mantra

I am positive.

Your own mantra(s):

I AM AGELESS NOW

date

day 21 **30-DAY TRANSFORMATION**

Today's suggested purposeful and intentional movement: Stretch the side of the hips (14) Bender Ball skater balance (21) Arm/shoulder strengthening with tube (32) Seated core with Bender Ball and tubing (37)

What else did you do? How did it make you feel?

Today's higher-level nutrition:

Mindful breathing and body scan:

HYDRATION

How old would you be if you didn't know how old you were?

Mantra

I am secure.

Your own mantra(s):

I AM AGELESS NOW

date day 22 **30-DAY TRANSFORMATION**

Today's suggested purposeful and intentional movement: Restore the neck (49) Restore the outer thigh (46) Restore the hamstrings (45) Restore the calves (40)

What else did you do? How did it make you feel?

Today's higher-level nutrition:

Mindful breathing and body scan:

HYDRATION

Eating good food doesn't have to suck.

Mantra

I am healthy.

Your own mantra(s):

I AM AGELESS NOW

date

day 23 **30-DAY TRANSFORMATION**

Today's suggested purposeful and intentional movement: Standing balance with tubing (36) Hand balance with Bender Ball (28) Side lying core with Bender Ball (26) Lunging with Gliding (16)

What else did you do? How did it make you feel?

Today's higher-level nutrition:

Mindful breathing and body scan:

HYDRATION

You're not
too old
and it's
never
too late.

Mantra

I am safe.

Your own mantra(s):

I AM AGELESS NOW

date day 24 **30-DAY TRANSFORMATION**

Today's suggested purposeful and intentional movement: Stretch the front of the hip (12) Plank with Gliding (18) Seated core with Bender Ball (25) Hip flexor stretch with Bender Ball (31)

What else did you do? How did it make you feel?

Today's higher-level nutrition:

Mindful breathing and body scan:

HYDRATION

Moving should be sustainable, and it will keep you younger longer than about any other practice.

Mantra

I am deserving.

Your own mantra(s):

I AM AGELESS NOW

date

day 25 **30-DAY TRANSFORMATION**

Today's suggested purposeful and intentional movement: Skater with Gliding (17) Plank with gliding (18) Side lying core (38) Seated core with Bender Ball and Gliding (37)

What else did you do? How did it make you feel?

Today's higher-level nutrition:

Mindful breathing and body scan:

HYDRATION

Wisdom is valuable. You've earned it with your experience. Age is the advantage.

Mantra

I am courageous.

Your own mantra(s):

I AM AGELESS NOW

date

day 26 **30-DAY TRANSFORMATION**

Today's suggested purposeful and intentional movement: Hand balance with Bender Ball (28) Side lying core with Bender Ball (26) Bender Ball squat with Balance (22) Bender Ball skater with Balance (21)

What else did you do? How did it make you feel?

Today's higher-level nutrition:

Mindful breathing and body scan:

HYDRATION

You may have spent the first half of your life trying to meet other people's expectations. The second half should be pure blue sky.

Mantra

I am desirable.

Your own mantra(s):

I AM AGELESS NOW

date

day 27 **30-DAY TRANSFORMATION**

Today's suggested purposeful and intentional movement: Bender Ball directional lunges (23) Bender Ball seated core (25) Bender Ball hands and knees balance (27) Balance and hamstring stretch with Bender Ball (30)

What else did you do? How did it make you feel?

Today's higher-level nutrition:

Mindful breathing and body scan:

HYDRATION

Be obsessed with being happy with your life, not with creating an image of what someone else thinks your life should be.

Mantra

I am talented.

Your own mantra(s):

I AM AGELESS NOW

date

day 28 **30-DAY TRANSFORMATION**

Today's suggested purposeful and intentional movement: Foot massage (1) Stretch the back of your hips (13) Stretch the side of your hips (14) Massage your glutes (4)

What else did you do? How did it make you feel?

Today's higher-level nutrition:

Mindful breathing and body scan:

HYDRATION

If you're stuck,
change your
mind,
If your past
is too painful,
move on.

Mantra

I am confident.

Your own mantra(s):

I AM AGELESS NOW

date

day 29 **30-DAY TRANSFORMATION**

Today's suggested purposeful and intentional movement: Lunging with Gliding (16) Bender Ball squat (22) Bender Ball directional lunges (23) Skater with Gliding (17)

What else did you do? How did it make you feel?

Today's higher-level nutrition:

Mindful breathing and body scan:

HYDRATION

Begin.

Begin again if you need to.

Trust yourself.

Mantra

I am Ageless Now.

Your own mantra(s):

date day 30 **30-DAY TRANSFORMATION**

Today's suggested purposeful and intentional movement: Massage the feet (1) Massage the hip flexors (5) Massage your forearms (10) Massage your neck (9)

What else did you do? How did it make you feel?

Today's higher-level nutrition:

Mindful breathing and body scan:

HYDRATION

I AM
AGELESS
NOW

iamagelessnow.com